GENERIC DRUGS: NEEDS AND ISSUES

HEALTH CARE ISSUES, COSTS AND ACCESS SERIES

The Health Care Financial Crisis: Strategies for Overcoming an "Unholy Trinity"
Cal Clark and Rene McEldowney (Editors)
2001. ISBN: 1-56072-924-4

Health Care Crisis in America
James B. Prince (Editor)
2006. ISBN: 1-59454-698-4

A New Epidemic: Harm in Health Care-How to Make Rational Decisions about Medical and Surgical Treatment
Aage R. Moller
2007. ISBN: 1-60021-884-9

Decision Making in Medicine and Health Care
Partricia C. Tolana (Editor)
2008. ISBN: 1-60021-870-9

Decision Making in Medicine and Health Care
Partricia C. Tolana (Editor)
2008. ISBN: 978-1-60692-561-4 (Online Book)

Social Sciences in Health Care and Medicine
Janet B. Garner and Thelma C. Christiansen (Editor)
2008. ISBN: 978-1-60456-286-6

Health Care Policies
Linda A. Bartlette and Ida F. Lawson (Editor)
2008. ISBN: 978-1-60456-352-8

Handbook of Stress and Burnout in Health Care
Jonathon R.B. Halbesleben (Editor)
2008. ISBN: 978-1-60456-500-3

GENERIC DRUGS: NEEDS AND ISSUES

RYAN S. BLANTON
EDITOR

Nova Science Publishers, Inc.
New York

NOTICE TO THE READER

LIBRARY OF CONGRESS CATALOGING-IN-PUBLICATION DATA

Generic drugs : needs and issues / editor, Ryan S. Blanton.
       p. ; cm.
 Includes bibliographical references and index.
 ISBN 978-1-60692-843-1 (hardcover)
 1. Generic drugs--United States. I. Blanton, Ryan S.
 [DNLM: 1.   Drugs, Generic--United States. 2.   Drug Industry--ethics--United States. 3. Government Regulation--United States. 4. Legislation, Drug--United States. QV 55 G3265 2009]
RS55.2.G465 2009
 338.4'76151--dc22
                                                                                2009027054

Published by Nova Science Publishers, Inc. ✝ *New York*

CONTENTS

PREFACE

The practice of "authorized generics" has recently been the subject of considerable attention by the pharmaceutical industry, regulators, and members of Congress alike. An "authorized generic" (sometimes termed a "branded," "flanking," or "pseudo" generic) is a pharmaceutical that is marketed by or on behalf of a brand name drug company, but is sold under a generic name. Although the availability of an additional competitor in the generic drug market would appear to be favorable to consumers, authorized generics have nonetheless proven controversial. Some observers believe that authorized generics potentially discourage independent generic firms both from challenging drug patents and from selling their own products. This book presents an analysis of the innovation and public health issues relating to authorized generic drugs. The book begins with a review of the procedures through which independent generic drug companies receive government permission to market their products and resolve patent disputes with brand-name firms. It also provides detailed background information pertaining to the concept of authorized generics and assesses their potential impact upon patent challenges and consumer welfare, as well as a summary of congressional issues and possible alternatives.

In: Generic Drugs: Needs and Issues
Editor: Ryan S. Blanton

ISBN: 978-1-60692-843-1
© 2009 Nova Science Publishers, Inc.

Chapter 1

AUTHORIZED GENERIC PHARMACEUTICALS: EFFECTS ON INNOVATION[*]

Congressional Research Service

SUMMARY

The practice of "authorized generics" has recently been the subject of considerable attention by the pharmaceutical industry, regulators, and members of Congress alike. An "authorized generic" (sometimes termed a "branded," "flanking," or "pseudo" generic) is a pharmaceutical that is marketed by or on behalf of a brandname drug company, but is sold under a generic name. Although the availability of an additional competitor in the generic drug market would appear to be favorable to consumers, authorized generics have nonetheless proven controversial. Some observers believe that authorized generics potentially discourage independent generic firms both from challenging drug patents and from selling their own products.

These perceived disincentives result from the provisions of the Drug Price Competition and Patent Term Restoration Act of 1984. Better known as the Hatch-Waxman Act, this legislation provides independent generic firms with a reward for challenging patents held by brand-name firms. That "bounty" consists of a 180-day generic drug exclusivity period awarded to the first patent challenger. During the 180-day period, the brand-name company and the first generic applicant are the only firms that receive authorization to sell that pharmaceutical. At the close of this period, other

---

[*] This is an edited, reformatted and augmented version of a Congressional Research Service publication, Report RL33605, updated January 10, 2008.

independent generic competitors may obtain marketing approval and enter the market, ordinarily resulting in lower prices for generic medicines.

Some commentators view the 180-day exclusivity period as a crucial incentive for generic firms to challenge patents held by brand-name firms. Under this view, the launch of an authorized generic during the 180-day exclusivity period makes the recovery of litigation expenses more difficult. In turn, the possibility that a brandname firm will sell an authorized generic during the 180-day exclusivity period may decrease the incentives of generic firms to challenge patents in the first instance.

Other observers believe that authorized generics benefit consumers by increasing competition in the generic market. Because the authorized generic is manufactured by the brand-name firm and identical to its own product, consumers may be encouraged to switch to the lower-cost authorized generic alternative. Authorized generics may also facilitate the settlement of patent litigation between brand-name and independent generic firms. As an historical matter, certain of these settlement agreements have allowed authorized generics to enter the market, and therefore promoted competition, prior to the expiration of the relevant patent term.

Recent judicial opinions have upheld FDA practices allowing authorized generics. As a result of congressional interest, however, the Federal Trade Commission has agreed to release a report directed towards this issue. Although Congress may wish to take no action if the current allowance of authorized generics is deemed appropriate, other possibilities include subjecting them to the 180-day generic exclusivity period enjoyed by an independent generic firm, or simply disallowing them altogether.

This report will be updated as needed.

AUTHORIZED GENERIC PHARMACEUTICALS: EFFECTS ON INNOVATION

Rising health care costs have for many years focused congressional attention upon the development and availability of prescription drugs. Recently, the presence of "authorized generic" pharmaceuticals in the drug marketplace has been the subject of congressional concern.[1] An "authorized generic" is a pharmaceutical that is marketed by or on behalf of a brand-named drug company, but is sold under a generic name. The brand-name firm may distribute the drug under its own auspices or via a license to a generic drug company. The price of

---

[1] *See* Thomas Chen (2007). Authorized Generics: A Prescription for Hatch-Waxman Reform, *Virginia Law Review*, *93*, 459; Saami Zain, (2007). Sword or Shield? An Overview and Competitive Analysis of the Marketing of 'Authorized Generics', *Food & Drug Law Journal, 62*, 739.

this "authorized copy" is ordinarily lower than that of the brand-name drug.[2] Some sources refer to authorized generics as "branded,""flanking," or "pseudo" generics."[3]

Authorized generics may be pro-consumer in that they potentially increase competition and lower prices, particularly in the short-term. They have nonetheless proven controversial. Authorized generics ordinarily enter the market at about the time the brand-name drug company's patents are set to expire.[4] Some observers argue that such products may possibly discourage independent generic firms both from challenging drug patents and from selling their own generic products.[5] The potential diminution in independent generic incentives may in turn lead to less desire on the part of brand-name firms to market authorized generics themselves.

This chapter presents an analysis of the innovation and public health issues relating to authorized generic drugs. The report begins with a review of the procedures through which independent generic drug companies receive government permission to market their products and resolve patent disputes with brand-name firms. It then provides detailed background information pertaining to the concept of authorized generics and assesses their potential impact upon patent challenges and consumer welfare. The report closes with a summary of congressional issues and possible alternatives.

MARKETING APPROVAL AND PATENT ISSUES FOR GENERIC DRUGS

The practice of authorized generics has arisen within a complex statutory framework established by the Drug Price Competition and Patent Term Restoration Act of 1984,[6] legislation more commonly known as the Hatch-

---

[2] *See* Leila Abboud (2004). 'Authorized Generics' Duel Grows, *Wall Street Journal* (March 25); Lcila Abboud, (2004). Drug Makers Use New Tactic to Ding Generic-Drug Firms, *Wall Street Journal* (January 27).

[3] *See* Blockbuster Drugs with Expiring Patents Gain New Hope: Generic Drugs, *Drug Week*, 352 (April 15, 2005).

[4] Stephen Barlas (2005). 'Authorized' Generics May Pose Unauthorized Problems: Government Worries About Potential Brand-Name Blocking Technique, *Pharmacy and Therapeutics*, 30, no.8, 435.

[5] *See* Michelle L. Kirsche (2005). Despite Challenges, Generics Dispensing is on the Rise, *Drug Store News*, 27, no. 4 at 20 (March 21).

[6] P. L. (1984). 84-417, *Stat.*, 98, 1585.

Waxman Act.[7] Under parameters established by that statute, a manufacturer that wishes to sell a generic drug must both obtain marketing approval from the Food and Drug Administration (FDA) and account for any patent rights that pertain to that product. This report first addresses FDA marketing approval procedures for generic drugs, and then turns to possible patent implications.

FDA Approval Procedures

The FDA regulates the marketing of pharmaceuticals in the interest of public health.[8] Under this regime, the developer of a new drug must demonstrate that the product is safe and effective before it can be distributed to the public. This showing typically requires the drug's sponsor to conduct both preclinical and clinical investigations.[9] In deciding whether to issue marketing approval or not, the FDA evaluates the test data that the sponsor submits in a so-called New Drug Application (NDA).

Prior to the enactment of the Hatch-Waxman Act, the federal food and drug law contained no separate provisions addressing marketing approval for independent generic versions of drugs that had previously been approved by the FDA.[10] The result was that a would-be independent generic drug manufacturer had to file its own NDA in order to sell its product.[11] Some independent generic manufacturers could rely on published scientific literature demonstrating the safety and efficacy of the drug by submitting a so-called paper NDA. Because these sorts of studies were not available for all drugs, however, not all independent generic firms could file a paper NDA.[12] Further, at times the FDA requested additional studies to address safety and efficacy questions that arose

---

[7] *See, e.g.,* Laura J. Robinson (2003). Analysis of Recent Proposals to Reconfigure Hatch-Waxman, *Journal of Intellectual Property Law, 11,* 47.

[8] CRS Report RL30989, *The U.S. Drug Approval Process: A Primer,* by Blanchard Randall IV.

[9] *See* G. Lee Skillington & Eric M. Solovy (2003). The Protection of Test and Other Data Required by Article 39.3 of the TRIPS Agreement, *Northwestern Journal of International Law and Business, 24,* 1.

[10] *See* Alfred B. Engelberg (1999). Special Patent Provisions for Pharmaceuticals: Have They Outlived Their Usefulness?, *IDEA: Journal of Law and Technology, 39,* 389.

[11] *See* James J. Wheaton (1986). Generic Competition and Pharmaceutical Innovation: The Drug Price Competition and Patent Term Restoration Act of 1984, *Catholic University Law Review, 34,* 433.

[12] *See* Kristin E. Behrendt (2002). The Hatch-Waxman Act: Balancing Competing Interest or Survival of the Fittest?, *Food and Drug Law Journal, 57,* 247.

from experience with the drug following its initial approval.[13] The result was that some independent generic manufacturers were forced to prove once more that a particular drug was safe and effective, even though their products were chemically identical to those of previously approved pharmaceuticals.

Some commentators believed that the approval of an independent generic drug was a needlessly costly, duplicative, and time-consuming process.[14] These observers noted that although patents on important drugs had expired, manufacturers were not moving to introduce independent generic equivalents for these products due to the level of resource expenditure required to obtain FDA marketing approval.[15]

In response to these concerns, Congress enacted the Hatch-Waxman Act, a statute that has been described as a "complex and multifaceted compromise between innovative and generic pharmaceutical companies."[16] Its provisions included the creation of two statutory pathways that expedited the marketing approval process for independent generic drugs. The first of these consist of Abbreviated New Drug Applications, or ANDAs. An ANDA allows an independent generic applicant to obtain marketing approval by demonstrating that the proposed product is bioequivalent to an approved pioneer drug, without providing evidence of safety and effectiveness from clinical data or from the scientific literature. The second are socalled § 505(b)(2) applications, which are sometimes still referred to as "paper NDAs." Like an NDA, a § 505(b)(2) application contains a full report of investigations of safety and effectiveness of the proposed product. In contrast to an NDA, however, a § 505(b)(2) application typically relies at least in part upon published literature providing pre-clinical or clinical data.

The availability of ANDAs and § 505(b)(2) applications often allow an independent generic manufacturer to avoid the costs and delays associated with filing a full-fledged NDA. They may also allow an independent generic

---

[13] *Id.*

[14] *See, e.g.,* Justina A. Molzon (1996). The Generic Drug Approval Process, *Journal of Pharmacy and Law, 5,* 275 ("The Act streamlined the approval process by eliminating the need for [generic drug] sponsors to repeat duplicative, unnecessary, expensive and ethically questionable clinical and animal research to demonstrate the safety and efficacy of the drug product.").

[15] *See* Jonathan M. Lave (2002). Responding to Patent Litigation Settlements: Does the FTC Have It Right Yet?, *University of Pittsburgh Law Review, 64,* 201 ("Hatch-Waxman has also increased the generic drug share of prescription drug volume by almost 130% since its enactment in 1984. Indeed, nearly 100% of the top selling drugs with expired patents have generic versions available today versus only 35% in 1983.").

[16] Natalie M. Derzko (2003). A Local and Comparative Analysis of the Experimental Use Exception — Is Harmonization Appropriate?, *IDEA: Journal of Law and Technology, 44,* 1.

manufacturer, in many cases, to place its FDA-approved bioequivalent drug on the market as soon as any relevant patents expire.[17]

As part of the balance struck between brand-name and independent generic firms, Congress also provided patent proprietors with a means for restoring a portion of the patent term that had been lost while awaiting FDA approval. The maximum extension period is capped at a five-year extension period, or a total effective patent term after the extension of not more than 14 years.[18] The scope of rights during the period of extension is generally limited to the use approved for the product that subjected it to regulatory delay.[19] This period of patent term extension is intended to compensate brand-name firms for the generic drug industry's reliance upon the proprietary pre-clinical and clinical data they have generated, most often at considerable expense to themselves.[20]

Resolution of Patent Disputes

In addition to being the holder of an FDA-approved NDA, the brand-name pharmaceutical firm may own one or more patents directed towards that drug product.[21] The product described by an independent generic firm's ANDA or § 505(b)(2) application may possibly infringe those patents should that product be approved by the FDA and sold in the marketplace. The Hatch-Waxman Act therefore establishes special procedures for resolving patent disputes in connection with applications for marketing generic drugs.

---

[17] *See, e.g.,* Sarah E. Eurek, (2003). Hatch-Waxman Reform and Accelerated Entry of Generic Drugs: Is Faster Necessarily Better?, *Duke Law and Technology Review*, (August 13, 2003), 18.

[18] 35 U.S.C. (2004). § 156(b).

[19] 35 U.S.C. (2004). § 156(b)(1).

[20] CRS Report RL30756, *Patent Law and Its Application to the Pharmaceutical Industry: An Examination of the Drug Price Competition and Patent Term Restoration Act of 1984 ("The Hatch-Waxman Act")*, by Wendy H. Schacht and John R. Thomas. CRS Report RL32377, *The Hatch-Waxman Act: Legislative Changes Affecting Pharmaceutical Patents*, by Wendy H. Schacht and John R. Thomas.

[21] Patents, which are administered by the United States Patent and Trademark Office (USPTO), provide their owner with the ability to exclude others from making, using, selling, offering to sell or importing into the United States the patented invention. 35 U.S.C. § 271(a) (2004). The term of the patent is ordinarily set at twenty years from the date the patent application was filed, 35 U.S.C. § 154 (2004), although pharmaceutical patents may be extended in order to compensate for a portion of the patent term that was lost during FDA marketing approval procedures. 35 U.S.C. § 156 (2004). Patent proprietors are permitted to file a civil suit in federal court in order to enjoin infringers and obtain monetary damages. 35 U.S.C. § 281 (2004). Although issued patents enjoy a presumption of validity, accused infringers may assert that the patent is invalid or unenforceable on a number of grounds. 35 U.S.C. § 282 (2004).

In particular, the Hatch-Waxman Act requires each holder of an approved NDA to identify patents it believes would be infringed if a generic drug were marketed before the expiration of these patents.[22] The FDA then lists these patents in a publication titled *Approved Drug Products with Therapeutic Equivalence Evaluations*, which is more commonly known as the "Orange Book."[23] Would-be manufacturers of independent generic drugs must then engage in a specialized certification procedure with respect to Orange Book-listed patents. An ANDA or § 505(b)(2) applicant must state its views with respect to each Orange Book-listed patent associated with the drug it seeks to market. Four possibilities exist:

(1) that the brand-name firm has not filed any patent information with respect to that drug;

(2) that the patent has already expired;

(3) that the generic company agrees not to market until the date on which the patent will expire; or

(4) that the patent is invalid or will not be infringed by the manufacture, use or sale of the drug for which the ANDA is submitted.[24]

These certifications are respectively termed paragraph I, II, III, and IV certifications.[25] An ANDA or § 505(b)(2) application certified under paragraphs I or II is approved immediately after meeting all applicable regulatory and scientific requirements.[26] An independent generic firm that files an ANDA or § 505(b)(2) application including a paragraph III certification must, even after meeting pertinent regulatory and scientific requirements, wait for approval until the drug's listed patent expires.[27]

The filing of an ANDA or § 505(b)(2) application with a paragraph IV certification constitutes a "somewhat artificial" act of patent infringement under the Hatch-Waxman Act.[28] The act requires the independent generic applicant to notify the proprietor of the patents that are the subject of a paragraph IV

---

[22] 21 U.S.C. (2004). § 355(c)(2).

[23] *See, e.g.,* Jacob S. Wharton, (2003). 'Orange Book' Listing of Patents Under the Hatch-Waxman Act," *St. Louis University Law Journal, 47,* 1027.

[24] 21 U.S.C. (2004). § 355(j)(2)(A)(vii).

[25] *See* Douglas A. Robinson, (2003). "Recent Administrative Reforms of the Hatch-Waxman Act: Lower Prices Now In Exchange for Less Pharmaceutical Innovation Later?," *Washington University Law Quarterly, 81,* 829.

[26] 21 U.S.C. (2004). § 355(j)(5)(B)(i).

[27] 21 U.S.C. (2004). § 355(j)(5)(B)(ii).

[28] Eli Lilly & Co. v. (1990). *Medtronic, Inc.,* 496 U.S. 1047, 15 USPQ2d 1121.

certification.[29] The patent owner may then commence patent infringement litigation against that applicant.

If the NDA holder demonstrates that the independent generic firm's proposed product would violate its patents, then the court will ordinarily issue an injunction that prevents the generic drug company from marketing that product. That injunction will expire on the same date as the NDA holder's patents. Independent generic drug companies commonly amend their ANDAs or § 505(b)(2) applications in this event, replacing their paragraph IV certifications with paragraph III certifications.[30]

On the other hand, the courts may decide in favor of the independent generic firm. The court may conclude that the generic firm's proposed product does not infringe the asserted patents, or that the asserted patents are invalid or unenforceable.[31] In this circumstance, the independent generic firm may launch its product once the FDA has approved its ANDA or § 505(b)(2) application. In addition, the independent generic firm may benefit from a 180-day period of marketing exclusivity, a concept this report describes next.

Generic Marketing Exclusivity

The Hatch-Waxman Act provides prospective manufacturers of independent generic pharmaceuticals with a reward for challenging the patent associated with an approved pharmaceutical. The reward consists of a 180-day generic drug exclusivity period awarded to the first ANDA applicant to file a paragraph IV certification. During this 180-day period, the FDA may not approve another ANDA containing a paragraph IV certification with respect to the same drug.[32] Notably, the 180-day generic drug exclusivity applies only to ANDA applicants, and not to those filing § 505(b)(2) applications.[33]

---

[29] 21 U.S.C. (2004). § 355(j)(2)(B)(i).

[30] 21 C.F.R. (2006). § 314.94(a)(12)(viii)(C)(1)(i).

[31] Although patents enjoy a presumption of validity, 35 U.S.C. § 282 (2004), that presumption is not uncontestable. Accused infringers may demonstrate that the patent does not meet the standards established by the Patent Act, and as a result should not have been issued by the U.S. Patent and Trademark Office. *Id.* In addition, an accused infringer may demonstrate that the patent is unenforceable on a number of grounds, among that its owner has engaged in "misuse" of the patent. *Id.*

[32] 21 U.S.C. (2004). §355(j)(5)(B)(iv).

[33] U.S. Dept. of Health and Human Services., Food and Drug Admin., Center for Drug Evaluation and Research, *Guidance of Industry, Listed Drugs, 30-Month Stays, and Approval of ANDAs*

Commentators have long referred to this provision as creating "generic exclusivity" or "180-day exclusivity."[34] As originally enacted, the Hatch-Waxman Act allowed the brand-name firm and the first independent generic applicant to share the market for the first 180 days of generic competition. At the close of this period, other independent generic competitors could receive FDA marketing approval. Because market prices often drop considerably following the entry of additional generic competition, the first independent generic applicant could potentially obtain more handsome profits than subsequent market entrants.[35]

Congressional enactment of the Medicare Modernization and Improvement Act of 2003[36] clarified that more than one patent challenger can enjoy "generic exclusivity," provided that certain conditions are met. Following the 2003 statute, all "first applicants" are potentially entitled to the 180-day generic exclusivity.[37] The statute defines the term "first applicant" to mean all applicants who, on the first day on which a substantially complete generic application with paragraph IV certification is filed, did themselves file a substantially complete generic application with a paragraph IV certification.[38] The statute therefore makes clear that multiple first applicants — that is to say, more than one generic that filed a paragraph IV generic application on the same day — may each enjoy "shared exclusivity."

The 180-day generic exclusivity period is intended to ameliorate collective action problems that may arise with regard to pharmaceutical patent challenges.[39] Stated less technically, an independent generic firm that challenges a patent must bear the expensive, up-front cost of litigation. If the independent generic firm is successful, however, the challenged patent is declared invalid with regard to the entire pharmaceutical industry. Any firm — not just the one who challenged the patent — could then introduce a competing product to the marketplace. Understandably, this forced sharing may undermine the incentives any one

---

and 505(b)(2) Applications Under Hatch-Waxman, As Modified by the Medicare Prescription Drug, Improvement, and Modernization Act of 2003, at 5 n.14 (October 2004).

[34] *See, e.g.,* Valerie Junod, (2004). Drug Marketing Exclusivity Under United States and European Union Law, *Food and Drug Law Journal*, 59, 479; Gerry J. Elman, FDA Approval of Generic Drugs: Instituting a First Successful Defense Requirement for Generic Exclusivity, *Biotechnology Law Reporter*, 22, 97 (April 2003); Frederick Tong, "Widening the Bottleneck of Pharmaceutical Patent Exclusivity," 24 *Whittier Law Review* (2003), 775.

[35] *See* Michael Bobelian, (1984). Act Led to a Boom in Prescription Drug Litigation, *New York Law Journal*, 1, 231, col. 3 (May 24, 2004).

[36] P. L. (2003). 108-173, 117 Stat. 2066.

[37] 21 U.S.C. (2004). §355(j)(5)(B)(iv)(I).

[38] 21 U.S.C. (2004). §355(j)(5)(B)(iv)(II)(bb).

[39] Mova Pharm. Corp. v. Shalala, 140 F.3d 1060, 1064 (D.C. Cir. 1998).

independent generic firm would possess to challenge a brand-name firm's patent. The award of 180 days of generic exclusivity is therefore intended to allow a successful patent challenger to capture an individual benefit for its effort, in turn encouraging such challenges in the first instance.[40]

THE CONCEPT OF AUTHORIZED GENERICS

Authorized Generics Practice

As noted previously, an "authorized generic" is a pharmaceutical that is marketed by or on behalf of a brand-name drug company, but is sold under a generic name.[41] Authorized generics are thus similar to "private label" products, which are manufactured by one firm but sold under the brand of another. Although private label products are commonplace in food, cosmetic, and other markets, they have only recently attracted attention in the pharmaceutical industry.[42]

Current interest in authorized generics is largely due to a shift in corporate strategies that has been traced to the early 1990's. Until that time, many entrants in the pharmaceutical industry engaged exclusively either in selling brand-name, innovative drugs, or in selling generic drugs. Several other brand-name firms began to market authorized generics shortly before patents on their products were due to expire. Among such products were Nolvadex® (tamoxifen), authorized by the Stewart Pharmaceutical Division of ICI Americas (now AstraZeneca) and sold by Barr Laboratories; Dyazide® (triamterene/hydrochlorothiazide), marketed by SmithKline Beecham Pharmaceuticals (now GlaxoSmithKline); and Ventolin® (albuterol), authorized by GlaxoSmithKline and sold by Dey LP.[43]

Many brand-name firms did not continue to sell authorized generics at that time, however, reportedly due to a lack of profitability.[44] One reason for the

---

[40] *See generally* Joseph Scott Miller, (2004). "Building a Better Bounty: Litigation-Stage Rewards for Defeating Patents," *Berkeley Technology Law Journal, 19,* 667.

[41] *See* Leila Abboud, (2004). 'Authorized Generics' Duel Grows, *Wall Street Journal* (March 25,); Leila Abboud, (2004). Drug Makers Use New Tactic to Ding Generic-Drug Firms, *Wall Street Journal* (January 27).

[42] *See* John Schmeltzer, (2006). Upscale Generics Make Gains: 'Private Label' Items Battling Brand Names, *Montgomery County Herald* (May 19).

[43] As brand-generic alliances grow, opponents cry foul, *Drug Store News* (August 23, 2004).

[44] Sanda Levy, "Why authorized generics are making a comeback," *Drug Topics: The Online Newspaper for Pharmacists,* available at [http://www.drugtopics.com/drugtopics/article/articleDetail.jsp?id=111159].

"resurgence" of authorized generics in the early 2000's is that physicians, pharmacists and patients more rapidly switch to generic drugs upon their introduction to the marketplace than a decade ago.[45] Because the rate of generic adoption is much greater now, brandname firms reportedly are more willing to "genericize" their own brands in order to capture a share of that market.[46] The expanding generic adoption rate has also reportedly led to an industry trend where brand-name houses acquire generic firms.[47] This development too may encourage authorized generics practice in the future.

In line with current trends, a number of successful paragraph IV ANDA applicants have faced competition from authorized generics during the 180-day generic exclusivity period. These independent generic firms include Barr, for the product Allegra® (fexofenadine);[48] Eon, for the product Wellbutrin SR® (bupropion SR);[49] and Teva, for the product Glucophage®.[50] Some industry analysts believe that authorized generics will form an increasingly prominent feature of the U.S. pharmaceutical market in the future.[51] Other commentators believe that this time has already arrived: According to one account, since 2004 "authorized generic versions have appeared for nearly all drugs with expiring U.S. patents."[52]

Authorized Generics within the Hatch-Waxman Framework

Authorized generics practice has proven controversial due to the Hatch-Waxman Act's architecture and incentive structures. Some commentators have voiced concerns that the introduction of authorized generics, particularly during the 180-day market exclusivity granted to the independent generic firm that brought a paragraph IV challenge, thwarts the policy goal of encouraging the

---

[45] *Id.*

[46] *Id.*

[47] *See* Andrew Humphries and Nick D'Amore, Generic Deluge: As U.S. Regulators Receive a Record Number of Generic Drug Applications, Pharmaceutical Companies Continue to Align With or Combat Generic Competition, 24 *Med Ad News*, no. 11 (November 1, 2005), 1.

[48] *See* Beth Understahl, (2005). Authorized Generics: Careful Balance Undone, *Fordham Intellectual Property, Media, and Entertainment Law Journal 16*, (Autumn), 355.

[49] *Id.*

[50] *See* Tara Croft, (2004). Building Teva, *Daily Deal* (October 25).

[51] *See* James Richie, (2006). Prasco's market share Rx: authorized generic drugs: Firm helps pharmaceutical companies retain profits, *Cincinnati Business Courier* (February 6).

[52] Tony Pugh, (2006). Drug companies battle generics with their own copies, *Duluth News-Tribune* (April 30).

introduction of generic pharmaceuticals.[53] In particular, critics argue that the use of authorized generics may discourage firms from filing paragraph IV patent challenges if their litigation expenses cannot be recouped through the 180-day market exclusivity period.[54] As antitrust attorney David A. Balto explains:

> The bounty from challenging a patent is very important. Pharmaceutical patent litigation is a multimillion-dollar proposition. But for the potential reward of sixmonth exclusivity that represents the vast majority of potential profits from generic entry, many firms might forgo challenging patents.[55]

For example, the FDA ruled that the generic manufacturer Apotex was entitled to 180-day exclusivity for its version of the anti-depressant drug Paxil® in 2003. The brand-name drug company, GlaxoSmithKline, introduced an authorized generic version of Paxil®. Although Apotex anticipated sales of up to $575 million during the 180-day generic exclusivity period, its sales were reported to be between $150 million and $200 million.[56] In a 2004 filing with the FDA, attorneys for Apotex asserted "that the authorized generic crippled Apotex's 180-day exclusivity — it reduced Apotex's entitlement to about two-thirds — to the tune of approximately $400 million."[57]

In addition, brand-name firms commonly introduce authorized generics on the eve of generic competition. Without an independent generic patent challenger in the first instance, brand-name firms may themselves make diminished, or delayed, use of the authorized generic strategy. As a result, the pro-competitive benefits of authorized generics may be postponed, or not realized at all, should independent generic rivals become less willing to challenge patents held by brand-name firms.[58]

On the other hand, authorized generics potentially offer several benefits both to drug companies and to consumers. Authorized generics are commonly less expensive than the brand-name drug. The introduction of an authorized generic

---

[53] *See* Understahl, *supra* note 48.

[54] Tony Pugh, (2006). Loophole may dampen generic-drug boom, *San Jose Mercury News* (May 3), A1.

[55] David A. Balto, (2006). We'll Sell Generics Too: Innovator drug makers are gaming the regulatory system and harming competition, *Legal Times*, no. 12, 39, (March 20, 2006).

[56] *See* Jenna Greene, (2006). The Drug Industry Has Figured Out a Way to Best Generic Competition, and Pharmaceutical Patent Litigation Could Free-Fall, *New Jersey Law Journal*, *183*, (January 23), 217.

[57] *See* Pugh, *supra* note 54.

therefore allows a lower-cost product to be made available to the consumer.[59] As the FDA opined in a statement issued in July 2004:

> Marketing of authorized generics increases competition, promoting lower prices for pharmaceuticals, particularly during the 180-day exclusivity period in which the prices for generic drugs are often substantially higher than after other generic products are able to enter the market.[60]

In addition, once a generic version of a drug becomes available following patent expiration, brand-name firms may lose considerable market share. Indeed, many health management organizations and insurance companies reportedly promote the use of generic substitutes for brand-name medications once they become available.[61] Absent participation in the generic market, brand-name firms may not be able to take advantage of investments they previously made with respect to their manufacturing facilities. Authorized generics therefore allow brand-name firms to continue to employ their manufacturing facilities at or near peak capacity even following patent expiration.[62]

Authorized generics may also support the research and development efforts of brand-name firms by providing them with additional revenue. Authorized generics may supply the brand-name firm with an additional income source, such as a royalty on sales made by its generic subsidiary or contracting partner.[63] These funds, or some portion of them, can potentially be employed in support of pharmaceutical innovation. Authorized generics may also facilitate settlement of patent infringement suits between brand-name and independent generic firms. A judicial holding of patent invalidity may have a severe impact upon a brand-name

---

[58] *See* Narinder Banait, (2005). Authorized Generics: Antitrust Issues and the Hatch-Waxman Act, Mondaq (November 4).

[59] Morton I. Kamien & Israel Zang, Virtual Patent Extension by Cannibalization, *Southern Economic Journal*, July 1999.

[60] U.S. Food and Drug Administration, *FDA Supports Broader Access to Lower Priced Drugs*, FDA Talk Paper, July 2, 2004. A study prepared by IMS Consulting for the Pharmaceutical Research and Manufacturers of America reached a similar conclusion, determining that the average price discount to brand-name drugs during the 180-day exclusivity period is greater when an authorized generic has been marketed than when one has not. IMS Consulting, *Assessment of Authorized Generics in the U.S.* (Spring 2006), available at [http://www.phrma.org/files/IMS%20Authorized%20Generics% 20Report_6-22-06.pdf].

[61] Kathleen Kerr, (2006). Prescription Hurdles: Need Brand-Name Drug? Generic May Come First, *Newsday* (March 16), B13.

[62] Jon Hess & Elio Evangelista, (2005). *Authorized Generics: Lifecycle Management's Compromise in the Patent Wars* (Cutting Edge Information, August 23), 4.

[63] *Id.*

firm in terms of its lost revenue. Many observers also believe that patent litigation is an uncertain venture.[64] By settling patent litigation, and allowing an ANDA applicant to produce an authorized generic, brand-name firms may potentially better manage risk. Such a technique provides a more stable revenue stream, both in support of the brand-name firm's research and development activities and for its investors. The generic company making an authorized generic can also benefit by not having to expend funds on litigation with an uncertain outcome or pursue an ANDA at the FDA, while expanding its product line, acquiring manufacturing experience, and gaining the firstmover advantage in the generic market.[65]

The use of authorized generics as a litigation settlement mechanism also impacts consumers, but in a manner that is both less certain and likely varies on a case-bycase basis. On one hand, particular settlement agreements may provide for the sale of authorized generics years before the disputed patent is set to expire. As a result, consumers may gain early access to a lower-cost alternative to the brand-name drug. On the other hand, had the generic firm refused to settle and ultimately prevailed in the litigation, then the market would have been open to full competition even earlier. The impact upon competition of a litigation settlement likely depends upon a number of complex factors, including the strength of the patent, the number of potential generic competitors, and the precise terms of the litigation settlement agreement.

Legality of Authorized Generics

The policy debate concerning authorized generics has been accompanied by legal challenges before the FDA and the courts concerning this practice. Opponents of authorized generics have contended that the Hatch-Waxman Act's generic exclusivity provisions should be understood as excluding authorized generics from the marketplace for the 180-day period.[66] The FDA has taken the opposite view, however, reasoning that the Hatch-Waxman Act does not require a brand-name pharmaceutical company to file any sort of application in order to

---

[64] *See* James Bessen & Michael J. Meurer, (2005). Lessons for Patent Policy from Empirical Research on Patent Litigation, *Lewis and Clark Law Review*, 9, 1.

[65] Christopher Worrell, (2004). *Authorized Generics*, presentation given at The 5th Generic Drugs Summit, September 27-29, and David Reiffen and Michael R. Ward, *"Branded Generics" as a Strategy to Limit Cannibalization of Pharmaceutical Markets*, May 2005, 2-4 available at [http://www.uta.edu/faculty/mikeward/brandedgenerics.pdf]

[66] *See* Generic Pharmaceutical Association, *Comment in Support of Citizen Petition Docket No. 2004P-0075/CP1* (May 21, 2004), available at [http://www.fda.gov/ohrms/dockets/dailys/04/June04/060404/04p-0075-c00003-vol1.pdf].

market the drug as an authorized generic.[67] In turn, the 180-day period of generic exclusivity provided by the Hatch-Waxman Act only applies to ANDA or § 505(b)(2) applications with paragraph IV certifications. As a result, the 180-day generic exclusivity period does not bar authorized generics from entering the market.

Two notable judicial opinions have recently upheld the FDA's position favoring authorized generics. In the first of these opinions, *Teva Pharmaceutical Industries, Ltd. v. Crawford*,[68] the Court of Appeals for the D.C. Circuit found no reasonable reading of the Hatch-Waxman Act that would allow authorized generics to be barred by the 180-day generic exclusivity period. In that case, independent generic manufacturer Teva had previously entered into an arrangement with Purepac Pharmaceutical Co., the first paragraph IV ANDA applicant with respect to the drug gabapentin. Teva and Purepac had agreed to share the 180-day generic exclusivity period. During that period, however, Pfizer sold its own authorized generic version of gabapentin, which was priced substantially below the price of its brand-name drug.[69]

Teva responded by petitioning the FDA to prohibit the marketing of authorized generic versions of gabapentin during the 180-day generic exclusivity period. Alternatively, Teva asserted that Pfizer should be required to file a supplemental NDA (sNDA) before selling an authorized generic.[70] According to Teva, the impact of the latter proposed ruling would lead to the same outcome as the first: Pfizer would be compelled to respect the 180-day generic exclusivity period established by the Hatch-Waxman Act.

The FDA denied the petition, resulting in a Teva lawsuit against the FDA. The district court confirmed the FDA's views, concluding that "[n]othing in the statute provides any support for the argument that the FDA can prohibit NDA holders from entering the market with [an authorized] generic drug during the exclusivity period."[71] Teva then appealed to the Court of Appeals for the D.C. Circuit, which affirmed.

Chief Judge Ginsburg began his opinion by observing that the Hatch-Waxman Act did not stipulate the manner in which the holder of an approved NDA must market its drug. Further, prior to the enactment of the Hatch-Waxman

---

[67] *See* M. Howard Morse & Richard E. Coe, (2006). Authorized Generics Are Good for You: Competition from drug pioneers shouldn't trouble the FTC, *Legal Times*, *29*, no. 15 (April 10, 2006).

[68] 410 F.3d 51 (D.C. Cir. 2005).

[69] *Id.* at 52.

[70] *Id.* at 52-53.

[71] Teva Pharm. Indus. v. FDA, 355 F.Supp.2d 111, 117 (D.D.C. 2004).

Act, nothing in the Food, Drug, and Cosmetic Act prevented the NDA holder from marketing an authorized generic. The D.C. Circuit thus saw the issue as whether it should "declare that a previously lawful practice became unlawful when the Congress passed a statute that said nothing about that practice."[72]

The Court of Appeals further rejected Teva's "functional" interpretation of the Hatch-Waxman Act. According to Teva, the practice of authorized generics had "developed only recently as a routine brand-name business strategy" and therefore had not been anticipated by Congress. Further, authorized generics practice severely diminished generic incentives to challenge pharmaceutical patents. According to Teva, then, "adhering to the 'literal' terms of the statute would lead to an absurd result, namely, that [the Hatch-Waxman Act] grants only a 'meaningless' exclusivity against subsequent ANDA filers rather than a 'commercially effective' exclusivity that runs against the NDA holder as well."[73]

The D.C. Circuit responded by reasoning that the balance between innovation and competition struck by the Hatch-Waxman Act was "quintessentially a matter for legislative judgment," such that "the court must attend closely to the terms in which the Congress expressed that judgment."[74] Here, Chief Judge Ginsburg reasoned, the statute was unambiguous. Although the Hatch-Waxman Act barred the approval of subsequent ANDAs for 180 days, the statutory language simply did not speak to marketing arrangements made by the holder of the approved NDA. The court of appeals further observed that, even in the event that an NDA holder authorized a generic, the 180-day exclusivity period continued to bar other firms from marketing a generic version of the drug. As a result, authorized generic practice hardly rendered the Hatch-Waxman Act's generic exclusivity provisions "meaningless."[75] In conclusion, because the Hatch-Waxman Act "clearly does not prohibit the holder of an approved NDA from marketing, during the 180-day exclusivity period, its own 'brand-generic' version of its drug," FDA practices concerning authorized generics were affirmed.[76]

A second judicial opinion, Mylan Pharmaceuticals, Inc. v. U.S. Food and Drug *Administration*,[77] also concluded that the Hatch-Waxman Act "does not grant the FDA the power to prohibit the marketing of authorized generics during

---

[72] 410 F.3d at 53.

[73] *Id.* at 54.

[74] *Id.*

[75] *Id.*

[76] *Id.* at 55.

[77] 454 F.3d 270 (4th Cir. 2006).

the 180-day exclusivity period ...."[78] That case involved the pharmaceutical nitrofurantoin, which is used to treat urinary tract infections. When the FDA approved a paragraph IV ANDA filed by Mylan Pharmaceuticals, Inc, to sell nitrofurantoin, NDA holder Proctor & Gamble Pharmaceuticals, Inc., licensed a third party generic firm to sell an authorized generic version of the drug. Mylan reportedly lost sales of "tens of millions" of dollars due to this arrangement.[79]

Mylan challenged the FDA approval of authorized generics practice before the U.S. District Court for the Northern District of West Virginia. Mylan appealed the district court's dismissal of its case to the Court of Appeals for the Fourth Circuit, which affirmed. Citing the D.C. Circuit's decision in *Teva v. Crawford* with approval, the Fourth Circuit similarly concluded that the statute clearly defined the 180-day exclusivity period only with respect to other paragraph IV ANDAs, not to authorized generics.[80] The Fourth Circuit therefore concluded that "[a]lthough the introduction of an authorized generic may reduce the economic benefit of the 180 days of exclusivity awarded to the first paragraph IV ANDA applicant, § 355(j)(5)(B)(iv) gives no legal basis for the FDA to prohibit the encroachment of authorized generics on that exclusivity."[81] As a result, the district court's judgment was affirmed.

It is possible to criticize the statutory construction of both *Teva v. Crawford* and *Mylan v. FDA*. In particular, neither court of appeals stressed that the Hatch-Waxman Act describes the 180-day time frame as an "exclusivity period."[82] The term "exclusivity" might be viewed as a curious drafting choice in view of the ruling that generic firms must potentially compete alongside authorized generics during the 180-day period.

On the other hand, the notion of "shared exclusivity" that arose following the Medicare Modernization Act amendments may be viewed as codifying congressional intent that multiple generic applicants may enter the market during the 180-day marketing exclusivity period.[83] In addition, many prescription drugs are available in a number of different dosage forms and strengths. Under current Hatch-Waxman Act practice, each strength and dosage form is considered a separate drug product for which a distinct generic applicant can qualify for 180-day exclusivity.[84]

---

[78] *Id.* at 271.

[79] *Id.* at 273.

[80] *Id.* at 275.

[81] *Id.* at 276

[82] 21 U.S.C. (2004). § 355(j)(5)(B)(iv).

[83] *See supra* notes 36-38 and accompanying text.

[84] *See* Apotex, Inc. v. FDA, 414 F. Supp. 2d 61, 64 (D.D.C. 2006).

As a result, the term "exclusivity" may be considered to have a particular meaning in the Hatch-Waxman Act — one that does not necessarily mean that independent generic firms will not face competition during the 180-day period even in the absence of authorized generics. Of course, these provisions may also impact the incentives that independent generic firms possess to challenge pharmaceutical patents.

In any event, *Teva v. Crawford* and *Mylan v. FDA* currently represent the law of the land. Absent further judicial developments or congressional activity, authorized generics will be judged as legitimate means for NDA holders to market their products under the Hatch-Waxman Act.[85]

The FTC Report

The Federal Trade Commission has become increasingly interested in authorized generics practice. Initially, the agency reportedly took the view "that authorized generic agreements are pro-consumer because they allow multiple generic entrants sooner."[86] Over the past several years, the FTC has either agreed to or has declined to challenge such arrangements.[87]

More recently, the FTC has expressed concerns about authorized generics practice. Jon Leibowitz, one of five FTC Commissioners, reportedly stated that "the introduction of an authorized generic will likely diminish incentives for generic firms to challenge patents and incur substantial development and litigation costs."[88] Although the commissioner was said to be skeptical that authorized generics practice violated the antitrust laws, he reportedly stated that he was "persuaded that authorized generics may have competitive implications that could upset the Waxman-Hatch balance."[89]

---

[85] *See generally* Thomas P. Noud & Paul T. Meiklejohn, (2005). The Developing Law of Pharmaceutical Patent Enforcement, *Journal of the Patent and Trademark Office Society, 87,* 921.

[86] "Bristol/Teva 'Authorized' Generic Agreement Approved By FTC,' (2004). *The Pink Sheet,* May 31, 7.

[87] *See, e.g.,* FTC Press Release, "With Conditions, FTC Allows Cephalon's Purchase of CIMA, Protecting Competition for Breakthrough Cancer Drugs" (August 9, 2004), available at [http://www.ftc.gov/opa/ 2004/08/cimacephalon.htm]; Advisory Opinion In the Matter of Bristol-Myers Squibb Co., Docket No. C-4076 (May 24, 2004), available at [http://www.ftc.gov/os/caselist/c4076/040525advisoryc4076.pdf].

[88] "FTC Is Urged to Examine Authorized Generics," *Chain Drug Review, 27, no. 10* (June 6, 2005), at 257.

[89] Senators Request FTC Study on Authorized Generics, (2005). *World Generic Markets* (May 31).

The FTC is currently considering the authorized generics issue at greater length. In response to a written request by three U.S. Senators, the FTC agreed to study "how competition between Paragraph IV generics and authorized generics during the 180-day exclusivity period has affected short-run price competition and long-run prospects for entry by Paragraph IV generics."[90] The FTC will also address the impact of generic drug entry on the price of pharmaceuticals.[91] The report is expected to be released during the 2008 calendar year.

Issues in Innovation, Competition and Public Health

Because authorized generics are a relatively recent phenomenon, economic and scholarly evaluation of their effect upon innovation, competition and public health has been relatively limited. Even the handful of academic commentary reveals differences of views over their significance. This report next reviews two leading working papers that reached different conclusions about the impact of authorized generics practice upon social welfare.[92]

Authorized Generics and Consumer Welfare

One recent working paper, Authorized Generic Drugs, Price Competition and *Consumers' Welfare*, was authored by Ernst R. Berndt, a member of the faculty of the MIT Sloan School of Management, and several individuals associated with the private firm Analysis Group, Inc.[93] The Berndt study concluded that "on balance

---

[90] FTC Chairman Deborah Majoras quoted in "Authorized Generics Noose Tightens With 'Best Price' Proposal, FTC Study," *The Pink Sheet* (November 14, 2005), 20.

[91] *Id.*

[92] Two other notable published reports were sponsored by trade associations. The Pharmaceutical Research and Manufacturers of American (PhRMA), which represents brand-name firms, sponsored a report stating that authorized generics practice benefited consumers. That report can be found at [http://www.phrma.org/files/IMS%20 Authorized%20Generics%20Report_6-22-06.pdf]. The Generic Pharmaceutical Association subsequently sponsored its own report, which "came up with drastically different results." *See* Generic Drug Industry Challenges PhRMA Authorized Generic Study," *FDA Week* (August 4, 2006). The report is available at [http://www.gphaonline.org/ AM/Template.cfm?Section=Home§ion=2006&template=/CM/ContentDisplay.cfm&Conte ntFileID=329]

[93] Ernst R. Berndt, Richard Mortimer, Ashoke Bhattacharjya, Andrew Parcee, & Edward Tuttle, (2005). Authorized Generic Drugs, Price Competition and Consumers Welfare (October 26), available at [http://www.aei.org/ docLib/20051103_GenericsDraft.pdf]. The authors of the

authorized generics are unlikely to harm competition and can indeed benefit consumers."[94] The authors initially observed that authorized generics may potentially improve consumer welfare in several respects. In particular, by introducing price competition, the authorized generic could reduce the average price of the drug and result in greater marketplace penetration.[95] Because an authorized generic is identical to the brand-name drug, consumers who are loyal to the brand-name drug may also be encouraged to switch to the lower-cost authorized generic alternative.[96]

According to the Berndt study, because numerous factors determine the profitability of generic drugs, the additional variable of authorized generics should not substantially impact the decision of an independent generic firm to file a paragraph IV ANDA. These factors include the possibilities that the independent generic firm was not the first paragraph IV applicant, that the FDA may not approve its ANDA, and that other independent generic firms may sell the identical drug at a different dosage level during the 180-day exclusivity period.[97] Because independent generic firms have traditionally filed paragraph IV ANDAs despite these risks, the authors reason that "it is not clear that one additional factor, authorized generic entry, is sufficient to discourage many patent challenges."[98] The report further observed that, even with the entry of an authorized generic into the relevant market, the expected profits may still suffice to induce patent challenges.[99]

The Berndt study additionally reported empirical findings that, although the 180-day exclusivity period significantly increased short-run generic-to-brand price ratios, it had scant impact upon long-run generic-to-brand price ratios. Stated differently, once multiple generic products enter the market, the historical existence of an earlier 180-day generic exclusivity period had little effect upon drug pricing. The authors conclude that "high generic penetration and low generic-to-brand price ratios are achieved in the long run regardless of whether successful paragraph IV certifications occurred."[100]

---

paper acknowledge the funding support of Johnson and Johnson, but further state that "The opinions expressed herein are those of the authors, and may not necessarily reflect those of the institutions with which they are affiliated, or of the research sponsor."

[94] *Id.* at 1.

[95] *Id.* at 16.

[96] *Id.* at 13.

[97] *Id.* at 14.

[98] *Id.*

[99] *Id.*

[100] *Id.* at 17.

The Berndt study further addressed the concern that authorized generics may potentially delay generic entry. According to the authors:

It has been argued that authorized generics will deter paragraph IV certifications and potentially delay generic entry. Most drugs, however, do not face a paragraph IV certification (historically only about 20 percent have). If the anticipation of authorized generic entry decreases incentives for paragraph IV certifications for the drugs that do face paragraph IV certification, it will do so in those cases with the least likelihood of success. As a result, generic entry will not be delayed for most drugs (if any).[101]

To elaborate on this latter point, the report reasoned that authorized generics may also lead to the salutary effect of reducing wasteful litigation. According to the authors, independent generics have prevailed in Hatch-Waxman Act litigation 42 percent of the time. As a result, the "paragraph IV certifications that may be deterred by the prospect of authorized generic entry would most likely have a lower likelihood of success than average."[102] Because such litigation is less likely to lead to improved consumer access to independent generic drugs, any potential discouragement of this litigation due to authorized generics practice is unlikely to impact competition and public health, the Berndt study explained.

Some of the contentions of the Berndt study may be subject to criticism. First, while it is true that the percentage of ANDAs with paragraph IV certifications is relatively low, that set of challenged patents are most likely the ones with sufficient sales to attract generic interest.[103] In turn, the challenged patents are likely to have a disproportionate impact upon public health. Second, although experience with authorized generics has thus far been limited, some commentators believe that this practice is growing.[104] If so, the marketplace presence of authorized generics may not amount merely to one risk among many, but rather a certainty.

Finally, although a successful patent challenge may not have much impact upon drug prices years after the patent was scheduled to expire anyway, such a

---

[101] *Id.* at 19.

[102] *Id.* at 15.

[103] *See* Kimberly A. Moore, "Worthless Patents," 20 *Berkeley Technology Law Journal* (2005), 1532 ("Whether a patent is likely to end up in litigation is indicative of the value of the patent to both the patent owner and competitors, since competitors are unlikely to infringe a patent of low value.").

[104] *See* George E. Jordan, (2005). Trade officials will study so-called authorized generics, *Star-Ledger* (November 10), 59.

challenge ordinarily allows generic competition to take place earlier than had the patent not been invalidated.[105] The judicial holding that a pharmaceutical patent is invalid has significant short- and medium-term consequences, including lower consumer expenditures on that medication but also the innovator's diminished ability to recoup research and development costs. Achieving the socially optimal balance between innovation and competition ultimately remains a difficult policy question that authorized generics practice renders even more complex.

Authorized Generics and Patent Challenges

A second recent working paper, "Branded Generics" As a Strategy to Limit *Cannibalization of Pharmaceutical Markets*,[106] was less sanguine about the marketplace impact of authorized generics practice than the Berndt study. As the authors, David Reiffin of the U.S. Commodity Future Trading Commission and Michael R. Ward, a member of the economics faculty of the University of Texas at Arlington, concluded:

> Under current [FDA] regulations, the branded firm is not prohibited fromproducing [an authorized] generic drug during the exclusivity period. As in the analysis above, the introduction of a branded generic drug will reduce the successful litigant's profits significantly, creating a duopoly, rather than a monopoly during the 180 day period. Thus, branded generic entry in Paragraph IV cases can dramatically change the incentives of generic firms, perhaps eliminating the incentive to litigate the validity of patents in some cases.[107]

---

[105] *See* Stephanie Greene, (2005). A Prescription for Change: How the Medicare Act Revises Hatch-Waxman to Speed Market Entry of Generic Drugs, *Journal of Corporate Law, 30,* 309.

[106] David Reiffin & Michael R. Ward, 'Branded Generics' As a Strategy to Limit Cannibalization of Pharmaceutical Markets" (May 2005), available at [http://www.uta.edu/faculty/mikeward/brandedgenerics.pdf].

[107] *Id.* at 28-29. Two other studies reached similar conclusions. One study, written by a member of the Department of Economics of the University of Calgary, concluded that authorized generic practice deterred market entry by independent generic firms within the Canadian pharmaceutical market. Aidan Hollis, (2003). The Anti-Competitive Effects of Brand-Controlled 'Pseudo-Generics' in the Canadian Pharmaceutical Market, *Canadian Public Policy, 29, no. 1,* 21. Another, authored by a member of the California Western School of Law faculty, concludes that "introduction of generics by brand name firms before patent expiration may be anticompetitive." Bryan A. Liang, "The Anticompetitive Nature of Brand Name Firm Introduction of Generics Before Patent Expiration," *The Antitrust Bulletin, 41,* (Fall 1996), 599.

In reaching this conclusion, Reiffin and Ward explained that relatively few authorized generics had been introduced in the United States. Because the decision of an independent generic firm to submit a paragraph IV ANDA occurs prior to patent expiration, the authors asserted that "it seems reasonable to assume that the branded firm's action in the instances in which it took place was not anticipated by independent generic producers at the time they began the ANDA process."[108] Their report therefore develops an economic model representing "a stylized version of [pharmaceutical] industry characteristics and economic intuition."[109]

Although the Reiffin and Ward model is complex, its analysis is founded upon the notion that earlier entry by a firm into a generic market implies greater economic rents for that firm.[110] Generic firms essentially compete to obtain the largest rents by being the first market entrant, followed by diminished rewards for achieving "second place," further diminished rewards for "third place," and so on as additional firms commence sales. The authors' analysis reveals several salient points about authorized generics practice. Under their model, the anticipated entry of authorized generics should "crowd out" more than one independent generic firm.[111] Second, the "primary effect of branded generic strategy is to transfer rents from the consumer to the patent holder."[112] Finally, the effect of authorized generics upon generic drug prices is, according to Reiffin and Ward, less significant for larger markets than smaller ones.[113]

Some of the reasoning of the Reiffin and Ward study also is not immune to criticism. The authors are undoubtedly correct that past experience with authorized generics may not suggest the future impact of this practice, given the reported "resurgence" of authorized generic introductions in recent years.[114] Nonetheless, at least with respect to some medications, there has been no shortage of firms willing to compete in generic markets despite knowledge of potential competition. For example, on June 9, 2004, the FDA authorized fourteen firms to market Bayer's Cipro® (cirprofoxacin).[115] Similarly, on July 29, 2004, thirteen firms received FDA approval to market generic versions of Pfizer's Diflucan®

---

[108] *Id.* at 5.

[109] *Id.* at 15.

[110] *Id.* at 15.

[111] *Id.* at 18.

[112] *Id.* at 27.

[113] *Id.* at 27.

[114] *Id.* at 27.

[115] *See* Dept. of Health and Human Services, U.S. FDA, Center for Drug Evaluation and Research, *Approvals — June 2004*, available at [http://www.fda.gov/cder/ogd/approvals /ap0604.htm].

(fluconazole).[116] Due to the possibility of "shared exclusivity" following enactment of the Medicare Modernization and Improvement Act of 2003,[117] the likelihood of multiple generic market entrants during the 180-day statutory period has in fact increased. Future experience will undoubtedly enrich economic understanding of the costs and benefits of authorized generic practice.

CONCLUDING OBSERVATIONS

Although Congress made significant amendments to the Hatch-Waxman Act as recently as 2003,[118] authorized generics were not subject to discussion at that time. The rise of this practice, as well as the vigor of the debate surrounding it, suggests both the pace of change within the industry and the prominence of the pharmaceutical industry within the national public health system.

As discussion of authorized generics continues, Congress may wish to have a sense of its legislative options. Should Congress conclude that authorized generics are appropriate, then it may simply take no action. The opinions of the D.C. and Fourth Circuits suggest that, as currently drafted, the Hatch-Waxman Act does not allow the FDA to restrict the ability of brand-name firms to sell or approve of authorized generics.[119] Absent legislative input, the FDA may be unlikely to alter its interpretation of the Hatch-Waxman Act in this respect in the future.

If Congress instead believes that authorized generics practice may instead disrupt the "bounty" system established by the Hatch-Waxman Act, one option is to require brand-name firms to file a supplemental NDA, or a similar application, with the FDA.[120] This filing would then place the brand-name firm in the same category as generic applicants who did not qualify as the first to file. In turn, the 180-day generic exclusivity period would then apply to the authorized generic. Alternatively, Congress could simply disallow authorized generics practice, at least during the 180-day generic exclusivity period.

---

[116] *See* Dept. of Health and Human Services, U.S. FDA, Center for Drug Evaluation and Research, *Approvals — July 2004*, available at [http://www.fda.gov/cder/ogd/approvals /ap0704.htm].

[117] *See supra* notes 36-38 and accompanying text.

[118] Medicare Modernization and Improvement Act, P.L. 108-173, 117 Stat. 2066 (2003).

[119] *See supra* notes 68-81 and accompanying text.

[120] This option is essentially the same as the one that Teva unsuccessfully argued before the Court of Appeals for the District of Columbia Circuit in the *Teva v. Crawford* case. *See supra* note 70 and accompanying text.

Notably, whether the 180-day generic exclusivity period strikes an appropriate balance between encouraging patent challenges and ensuring prompt access to generic medications is itself a contested proposition within the pharmaceutical industry.[121] Discussion of the authorized generics issue may also prompt further reflection on the basic structure of incentives within the Hatch-Waxman Act.

Current interest in authorized generics reflects longstanding congressional concern for the appropriate balance between innovation and competition within the pharmaceutical industry. Although academic inquiry into authorized generics practice remains in its early phases, it is notable that knowledgeable commentators have reached disparate views of the benefits or detriments of this practice. Some observers stress that authorized generics benefit consumers by providing enhanced access to lower-cost alternatives to branded drugs, while others express concerns that authorized generics will defeat the incentives that independent generic firms possess to challenge pharmaceutical patents. The analysis to be provided in the forthcoming FTC report and other studies may shed additional light on the impact of authorized generics upon consumer welfare.[122]

---

[121] Letter of Robert A. Armitage, Eli Lilly & Company, Re: Authorized Generic Study (June 5, 2006), available at [http://www.ftc.gov/os/ comments/genericdrugstudy3/060605lilly.pdf].

[122] *See supra* notes 85-86 and accompanying text.

In: Generic Drugs: Needs and Issues
Editor: Ryan S. Blanton

ISBN: 978-1-60692-843-1
© 2009 Nova Science Publishers, Inc.

Chapter 2

PAYING OFF GENERICS TO PREVENT COMPETITION WITH BRAND NAME DRUGS: SHOULD IT BE PROHIBITED?[*]

OPENING STATEMENT OF HON. PATRICK J. LEAHY, A U.S. SENATOR FROM THE STATE OF VERMONT

Chairman LEAHY. Good morning. This hearing today is the continuation of a longstanding, bipartisan effort by several members of this Committee to provide consumers more choices and lowercost medicines. My focus is on making lower-cost generic medicines available not only to our families but to our seniors. The existing law is being misused by some brand-name and generic drug companies. The fact we have scheduled this hearing so early in this new Congress is a sign, I hope, that people realize that this is going to be a high priority for this Committee. It deserves to be and consumers want it to be.

We will examine the harmful effects of a type of collusion that limits consumer choices and that keeps consumer prices artificially high. Now, rarely do we have such a clear-cut opportunity to remove impediments that prevent competition and keep the marketplace from working as they should, to benefit consumers. Basically, as you know, we have had the situation where a drug company will actually pay a generic producer not to put a drug on the market so that they can keep the prices high.

---

[*] This is an edited, reformatted and augmented version of Senate Hearing 110-4 before the Committee on the Judiciary United States Senate, One Hundred Tenth Congress, First Session, on January 17, 2007, Serial No. J-110-4.

Now, Congress never intended for brand-name drug companies to be able to pay off generic companies not to produce generic medicines. We never intended that. That would be a sham, it would be harmful to consumers, and it would be a crime.

In fact, the history and text of the Hatch-Waxman laws make it clear that the opposite of delay was the goal.

Now, it is no secret that prescription drug prices are rising. They are a source of considerable concern to many Americans, especially senior citizens and working families. In a marketplace that is free of manipulation—free of manipulation—generic drug prices can be as much as 80 percent lower than the comparable brand-name version.

In June of last year, I sponsored a bill that was introduced by Senator Kohl of Wisconsin, also sponsored by Senators Grassley, Schumer, Feingold, and Johnson, which would have stopped these payoffs to delay access to generic medicines. Working with Senators Kohl and Grassley and with many others, we will try to enact a new version.

You know, it is unfortunate we even have to do this. As I said in June, there are still some companies driven by greed that may be keeping low-cost, life-saving generic drugs off the marketplace, off pharmacy shelves, and out of the hands of consumers by carefully crafted anticompetitive agreements.

Since some of these deals used to be done in secret, behind closed doors, I am glad that because of a bill that was reported out of this Committee, Congress is now aware of this problem. In 2001, I worked with Chairman Hatch and later with Senator Grassley to make sure that our law enforcement agencies—the Federal Trade Commission and the Department of Justice—at least were made aware of the secret, sometimes potentially criminal deals.

The New York Times and others published major investigative stories on how the manufacturer of a hypertension drug used to help prevent strokes and heart attacks—Cardizem CD—had made deals to pay a potential generic competitors $10 million every 3 months to stop it from developing a generic version of Cardizem. Of course they did. They were making a fortune, and they did not want those people who needed that drug to be able to buy a lowercost generic. This led to my introduction of S. 754, the Drug Competition Act, which was reported out of this Committee and was finally passed as part of the Medicare Modernization Act Amendments with significant help from Senator Grassley.

The concept of that law is simple: It requires if a brand-name company and a generic firm enter into an agreement that is related to the sale of either the brand-name drug or its generic version, then both companies must file copies of any agreements with the FTC and with the Department of Justice so those agencies can enforce the law. Incidentally, once the Cardizem deal was exposed and challenged, the U.S. Circuit Court held that the ''horizontal market allocation agreement...[was] per se illegal under the Sherman Act.''

Now, Commissioner Leibowitz will testify about what the FTC has found regarding these deals—the deals between the brandname companies and generic companies.

I will once again strongly support a legislative effort led by Senator Kohl and Senator Grassley to allow the FTC to do its job. Two subsequent circuit court decisions have undermined the Cardizem approach and relied on the general rule favoring settlements between private litigants, even though private corporate litigants have duties to their shareholders, not consumers, to maximize profits. The problem with respect to deals not to compete is that the interests of millions of senior citizens, millions of children, and millions of others are not taken into account. Those cases ignore the decision in Associated General in which the U.S. Supreme Court noted that ''the Sherman Act was enacted to assure our customers the benefits of price competition....'' The focus is on consumers, not on whether private companies should be able to make back-room deals that harm consumers as part of a settlement of a lawsuit.

Our bipartisan bill will solve that problem by making payments by brand-name companies to delay introduction of a generic drug unlawful. My initial position is to follow this bright-line approach. I will be interested in hearing from others, of course, and it will be a major priority of this Committee.

[The prepared statement of Senator Leahy appears as a submission for the record.] With that, I would yield to the distinguished senior Senator from Pennsylvania.

STATEMENT OF HON. ARLEN SPECTER, A U.S. SENATOR FROM THE STATE OF PENNSYLVANIA

Senator SPECTER. Thank you, Mr. Chairman.

This Judiciary Committee is used to hearings on important competing values and complex conceptual matters, and today's hearing is a top-drawer illustration of the issues which we confront and which are confronted here.

We have two very important values at issue here. One is to encourage pharmaceutical companies to develop life-saving drugs, and I can speak with some authority personally on that subject, having been the beneficiary of some very important drugs in battling Hodgkin's. Every 2 weeks I got a cocktail—not the kind of cocktail I would prefer. It was in the morning, and I did not like the ingredients, but it was life-saving. And the pharmaceutical companies take a decade or so to develop these drugs at a cost in the range, reportedly, of $1 billion. And only one out of thousands make it. They have a patent period no longer than 20 years to encourage them to develop further life-saving drugs. That is one very important value. On the other side of the issue is the matter of holding down costs so that these life-saving drugs in generic form can be available to more people to save their lives.

There are three studies which I think are worth noting at the outset of our hearing. One is a study, published by the Food and Drug Administration in 2005, that determined that once generics begin competing, prices fall by almost 50 percent. Second, according to the Generic Pharmaceutical Association, generic drugs account for 56 percent of all drug sales in the United States, while revenues from generic drugs are only one-tenth that of brand-name manufacturers. A third study, Pharmaceutical Care Management Association recently published findings that Medicare would save over $23 billion between now and 2010 by purchasing newly available generic drugs instead of the brand-name drugs that are currently purchased.

In my capacity as Chairman of the Appropriations Subcommittee dealing with the Department of Health and Human Services, I can attest to the grave difficulties of finding funding for very important medical matters like the National Institutes of Health and the Centers for Disease Control so that we deal with these kinds of savings that are very, very important.

The legal issues here are conceptually very complicated. We have had one circuit court, the Sixth Circuit, conclude that these settlement agreements are so-called per se antitrust violations. That is fancy Latin for meaning all you have to show is the settlement agreement and there is a violation of the antitrust laws. Two other circuits—the Second and the Eleventh Circuit—have said that a rule of reason applies, so it is a balancing test. And the articulated rule of reason is this: that patent settlements are reasonable so long as the exclusionary effects of the settlement do not exceed the exclusionary effects of the patent.

I do not think this hearing will be quite long enough to determine what that succinctly stated formula means. I have an expert in antitrust law, Ivy Johnson, and she has been trying to explain it to me for several days. And I have had experience in the antitrust field in the private practice of law before coming to the Senate and considerable experience here on this Committee.

In reviewing the leading cases, *Cardizem*, where the Sixth Circuit said it was a per se violation, and *Valley Drugs* and *Schering-Plough*, where the Eleventh Circuit said it was rule of reason, and the *Tamoxifen* case, where the Second

Circuit said it was rule of reason, involve extraordinarily complicated factual situations. One idea which occurs to me is whether when the lawsuits are settled where there is litigation between the generic maker and the patent holder, a condition of the settlement ought to be for the presiding judge to examine it and see if the settlement does or does not violate the antitrust laws, instead of inviting a later lawsuit where purchasers want lower costs and come in and sue the parties to the agreement.

The distinguished representative from the Federal Trade Commission, who performed—he just raised his eyebrows. You must agree with that—a lot of service for this Judiciary Committee and for Senator Kohl's Subcommittee, is going to testify, according to his written presentation, that there ought to be a per se violation. And the thought crosses my mind, if the FTC thinks that, why doesn't the FTC act on it?

There is a gesture of ''Who knows?'' And maybe it is more appropriately left to the Congress. Sometimes the gestures and the body language tell more than the long, verbose written and oral statements.

But as I look at this field, it is fraught with complexity on the competing values and fraught with complexity on what the parties have entered into. And I do think there is a burden on people making these settlements to show that they are not anticompetitive, because why settle the case unless it is in the advantage of the patent holder and raises a question which I am not prepared to answer: Is the generic company being bought off to the detriment of the public? But I commend the distinguished Chairman for convening this hearing and the work that Senator Kohl has done, and I regret that I am going to have to excuse myself early to attend a meeting by the National Security Counselor, who has invited a group of Senators to meet on the Iraq issue. We are being buffeted on all sides by complex issues.

Thank you, Mr. Chairman.

Chairman LEAHY. Thank you, Senator Specter, and I appreciate your being here for this because this will be a priority.

Before introducing Commissioner Leibowitz and swearing him in, I did want to yield to Senator Kohl, who will also take over and chair this hearing when I have to leave for another one of those similar kinds of things. There seems to be a lot of discussion in Washington about the war in Iraq of late, and I think that is a very good thing.

Senator Kohl?

STATEMENT OF HON. HERB KOHL, A U.S. SENATOR FROM THE STATE OF WISCONSIN

Senator KOHL. I thank you, Mr. Chairman, for calling this hearing here today. This hearing will examine legislation that you and I have sponsored, along with Senators Grassley and Schumer, that will end an anticompetitive abuse which denies millions of consumers access to generic drugs. Our bill does this by forbidding the collusive payoffs between brand-name drug companies and generics which are designed to keep low-cost alternatives off the market.

As health care costs continue to spiral upwards, the high price of prescription drugs leads the way. A recent independent study found that prescription drug spending has more than quadrupled since 1990. One way to tame the cost of prescription drugs is to promote the introduction of generic alternatives. Consumers realize substantial savings once generic drugs enter the market. One study estimates that every 1-percent increase in the use of generic drugs could save $4 billion annually in health care costs in our country.

Unfortunately, recent years have seen the growing practice of collusion between some brand-name drug manufacturers and generic manufacturers to prevent competition. This collusion consists of payments, often as much as hundreds of millions of dollars, made by brand-name companies to generic companies to settle patent litigation. In return for this money, the generic company promises to keep its competing drugs off the market. The brand-name company profits so much by delaying competition that it can easily afford to pay off the generic company. The losers, of course, are the American people who continue to pay unnecessarily high drug prices for years to come.

Just two examples of the benefits of early generic entry prior to patent expiration. No. 1, the generic version of Prozac, which entered the market in 2001, approximately 3 years before the patent expired, resulted in consumer savings of about $2.5 billion. No. 2, generic competition to Paxil in 2003, 3 years before the last patent would have expired, saved consumers about $2 billion.

The patent settlements targeted by our bill would eliminate such practices. The FTC has found that these agreements violate antitrust law. However, two circuit court decisions in 2005 allowed these agreements, regardless of their obvious anticompetitive impact, and the effect of these court decisions has been stark. In the year after these decisions, the FTC has found half of all patent settlements, 14 of 28, did involve payments from the brand-name to generic manufacturer in return for an agreement by the generic manufacturer to keep its drug off the market. In the year before these decisions, not a single patent settlement reported to the FTC contained such an agreement.

So I believe the time has now come to forbid these anticompetitive, anticonsumer, reverse payment patent settlements. The bill that we are introducing today does just that. It will state clearly and simply that it is unlawful under the antitrust laws for any drug maker to settle patent litigation by paying off a competitor in return for an agreement to keep a competing product off the market.

So I urge my colleagues to join us in supporting this legislation to end this anticompetitive practice that enriches drug companies at the expense of consumers. Offering consumers generic alternatives is essential to bringing high drug prices down, and we ought to have zero tolerance for efforts by big brand-name drug companies to pay off their competitors to keep competition off the market. These payoffs help big drug companies maximize their profits while ordinary consumers pay the price.

I am very pleased that we have a distinguished group of witnesses here today, and we are looking forward to their testimony.

Thank you, Mr. Chairman.

Chairman LEAHY. Thank you, Senator Kohl. And I know our first witness, Commissioner Leibowitz of the Federal Trade Commission, has had a long and distinguished public service. He was Democratic chief counsel and staff director for the U.S. Senate Antitrust Subcommittee from 1997 to 2000. He served as chief counsel and staff director for the Senate Subcommittee on Terrorism and Technology from 1995 to 1996 and the Senate Subcommittee on Juvenile Justice from 1991 to 1994. And very important to this Committee, he served as chief counsel to Senator Herb Kohl from 1989 to the year 2000. In the private sector, Mr. Leibowitz served most recently as vice President for Congressional affairs for the Motion Picture Association of America from 2000 to 2004. He is a Phi Beta Kappa graduate of the University of Wisconsin with a B.A. in American History, and he also graduate from the New York University School of Law in 1984.

Mr. Leibowitz, would you please stand so I can swear you in? Do you swear that the testimony you are about to give is the truth, the whole truth, and nothing but the truth, so help you God?

Mr. LEIBOWITZ. I do.

Chairman LEAHY. Thank you. And, Mr. Leibowitz, please go ahead with your testimony. I am going to switch seats with Senator Kohl because I will be leaving shortly after you finish.

STATEMENT OF JON LEIBOWITZ, COMMISSIONER, FEDERAL TRADE COMMISSION, WASHINGTON, D.C.

Mr. LEIBOWITZ. Thank you, Mr. Chairman.

Chairman Leahy, Ranking Member Specter, Senator Kohl, Senator Cardin, other members of the Committee, we applaud your early hearing on legislation to ensure that consumers continue to have access to low-priced generic drugs. It is critical to eliminate the pay-for-delay settlement tactics employed by the pharmaceutical industry. Simply put, companies should not be able to play ''Deal or No Deal'' at the expense of American consumers.

Mr. Chairman, I am particularly honored to return to the Committee for which I worked for so many years. In the introduction, you made me sound much more impressive than I know myself to be, but I do appreciate it. I am honored to come back here.

But let me start with the usual disclaimer. The written statement that we submitted represents the views of the Commission. My oral testimony reflects my own views, and not necessarily the views of any other Commissioner.

There is a particular urgency to pharmaceutical competition issues today. Recent appellate decisions make it difficult to challenge so-called exclusion payments—that is, patent settlements in which the brand-name drug firm pays the generic firm to stay out of the market. If these decisions are allowed to stand, drug companies will enter into more and more of these agreements, and prescription drug costs, which slowed in 2005 after years of precipitous growth, will begin to rise again. These increased costs will burden not only individual consumers, but also the Federal Government's new Medicare program, State governments, and American businesses striving to compete in a global economy—like General Motors, which reports that employee health care costs add $1,500 to the price of each and every car that rolls off its assembly line.

Mr. Chairman, as our 2006 Patent Settlement Report released today confirms, this is not just a theoretical concern. In the past year, we have seen a dramatic increase in these types of settlements.

Now, when Congress enacted the Hatch-Waxman statute in 1984, you encouraged speedy introduction of generics by establishing mechanisms to challenge invalid or narrow patents on branded drugs. This statutory framework ensures that our pioneer drug firms remain the envy of the world—and they are— while also delivering enormous consumer savings. When the first generic enters the market, it generally does so at a 20- to 30-percent discount off of the brand price. Prices drop even further, by 80 percent or more, after other generic competitors go to market, usually 6 months later. Generic competition following successful patent challenges in just four products—and, Senator Kohl, you alluded to some of these—Prozac, Zantac, Paxil, and Platinol—is estimated to have saved consumers more than $9 billion alone.

But these benefits will be at risk, as will the legacy of Hatch-Waxman itself, if companies are able to settle litigation through arrangements in which brands can pay generics to sit it out. Sadly, the incentives to enter into such pernicious pay-for-delay agreements are substantial because generic entry causes the branded drug firm to lose far more in sales than the lower-priced generic could ever possibly earn. As a result, with these agreements both firms are better off than they would be if they competed. Of course, consumers are left holding the bag or, more appropriately, footing the bill.

For the past decade, the FTC has made challenging these pharmaceutical patent settlements a bipartisan priority. In 2000 and 2001, the Commission obtained two major consents involving anticompetitive payments between brands and generics. We put companies on notice that we would consider all available remedies, including disgorgement of profits, against this behavior in the future, and our actions stopped this conduct cold.

The Commission set forth rules that everyone understood. If you settle a case by paying off a generic to stay out of the market, we will not let you get away with it. As a result, to the best of our knowledge, there were plenty of settlements between 2000 and 2004 and no exclusion payments.

In 2003, the Commission ruled that a 1997 settlement with a payment from Schering-Plough, which is the brand, to Upsher-Smith, the generic, violated the antitrust laws. The case involved a potassium supplement widely used by older Americans taking medication for high blood pressure. The Eleventh Circuit reversed us in 2005, and the Second Circuit, in a 2–1 decision in the *Tamoxifen* case, which Senator Specter alluded to, issued a similar holding later that year. These decisions, which essentially allow a patent holder to compensate a generic except under very limited circumstances, have dramatically altered the legal landscape—and, we believe, to the detriment of consumers.

Mr. Chairman, how do we know this to be accurate? Well, thanks to the reporting requirement that you, Senator Leahy, and Senator Grassley included in the 2003 Medicare Modernization Act, the FTC reviews each and every Hatch-Waxman settlement. Tellingly, here is what the data for the last few years reveals.

As you can see from the chart, for fiscal year 2004 and the early part of fiscal year 2005, none of the nearly 20 agreements reported between brands and generics contained both a payment from the brand and an agreement by the generic to defer entry. In other words, the parties could—and they did—settle patent litigation without money flowing to the generic.

But data from fiscal year 2006 is far more disturbing. The report that we released this morning shows that half of all settlements, 14 out of 28, involve some form of compensation to the generic and an agreement by the generic not to market its product for a period of time. Almost all the settlements with first filers, 9 out of 11, involve similar restrictions. In other words, just before *Schering* and *Tamoxifen*, there were no such payments. Just after these decisions, it appears to be the new way of doing business.

Mr. Chairman, given how profitable these agreements are for both the brands and the generics, it is not surprising that the industry has reacted so quickly to recent court decisions. After all, they do have responsibilities to their shareholders. Nor should it be hard to predict what will happen if nothing changes. There will be more and more of these settlements with later and later entry dates. No longer will generic companies vie to be the first to bring a drug to market. Instead, they will vie to be the first to be paid not to compete.

From our perspective, we will continue to be vigilant in looking for ways to challenge anticompetitive settlements. It is a matter of public knowledge that we are looking to bring a case that will create a clearer split in the circuits and encourage the Supreme Court to resolve this issue. But that could take years and the outcome is uncertain.

A legislative approach could provide a swifter, more certain, and more comprehensive solution. For that reason, we strongly support legislation to prohibit these anticompetitive payments, and we strongly support the intent of the bipartisan bill to be introduced by Senators Kohl, Leahy, Grassley, and others, which takes a bright-line approach to prohibiting these deals. Drafting such a measure is challenging. The deals are obviously very difficult or complex, so we are happy to work with you as the bill moves forward.

Mr. Chairman, we do have enormous respect for the pharmaceutical industry, both brands and generics. Brand drug companies pursue hundreds, perhaps thousands, of unsuccessful candidates for each one that comes to market, and these companies have brought significant health benefits to consumers—as Senator Specter said, life-saving drugs. For their part, generic drug companies have produced low-cost pharmaceuticals and pushed the brands to innovate even further and faster. And we are not opposed to all settlements. Let me try to briefly dispel that urban myth. We have brought only a handful of cases involving pharmaceutical agreements and none involving deals between 2000 and 2005— that is, before the *Schering* decision. But we do not and we cannot support settlements when brands and generics resolve their disputes at the expense of consumers.

Mr. Chairman, at a time when our Nation faces the challenge of rising health care costs, the antitrust laws and the Hatch-Waxman Act should be used to ensure innovation and lower prices. They should not be used to undermine competition, nor to evade congressional intent—though, of course, ultimately that is for you to decide.

Thank you so much. I am happy to answer questions.

Chairman LEAHY. I will be leaving now, as I said, turning over to Senator Kohl. I will submit some questions for the record. I am especially interested in your views on why the Justice Department declined the FTC's request on cert. after *Schering-Plough* to find out—to get some clarity. I would have thought that clarity would be in the interest of all of us, and I was surprised that they did not agree with you on that.

So, Senator Kohl, thank you very much.

Mr. LEIBOWITZ. Thank you, Senator.

Senator KOHL [PRESIDING.] Thank you, Chairman Leahy.

Commissioner Leibowitz, patent settlements between brandname and generic drug manufacturers in which brand-name companies pay generic companies many millions of dollars to keep their product off the market, how does this harm consumers? And are you in a position to quantify in any way the amount of higher drug prices that consumers have had to pay as a result of some of these settlements?

Mr. LEIBOWITZ. Well, there was a CBO study from 1994 that said consumers save $8 to $10 billion a year from generic drugs. But now there are many, many more generics on the market, many more drugs on the market, and so we think the savings are substantially greater.

It is hard to quantify the harm that we see from what we believe are these anticompetitive exclusion payments, but what they tend to do, essentially, the brand will pay the generic some form of consideration —it could be a cash payment; it could be not offering an authorized generic; it could be a licensing deal—and the generic will stay out of the market longer. It will not enter sooner. And the longer it stays it out of the market, of course, the more consumers are forced to pay higher prices for their drugs.

There is a huge incentive, obviously, to make these deals because the price goes down so much after the first generic and, really, subsequent generics enter. So there is always really a large ''sweet spot'' where the brand can pay the generic and the generic will earn more by not competing than by competing. And the brand will earn more by not having competition in the market, notwithstanding it has made this reverse payment.

Senator KOHL. Potentially, what will happen to the whole generic movement, in your opinion, if brand-name manufacturers are in a position to pay off generics to keep their product off the market and recognize how profitable this is to them, this whole generic movement which is saving consumers so much money, what will happen to it?

Mr. LEIBOWITZ. Well, I don't think you will see the end to the generic industry. Obviously, there are a number of generic drugs—hundreds, thousands— that are already out there. But what you would see is generic entry will be pushed back to the end of the patent of the brand—or 6 months before the patent of the brand—so it can retain that exclusivity. And I do not believe—although, again, this is for the three of you and the Committee to decide—we do not believe that that was the intent of Hatch-Waxman. The intent of Hatch-Waxman was to allow generics—when they were not infringing on the patent, or if the patent of the brand was invalid—to enter the market sooner and to bring these low-cost drugs to consumers.

Senator KOHL. Thank you.

Senator Specter, do you have questions?

Senator SPECTER. Yes, thank you very much, Mr. Chairman.

Commissioner Leibowitz, is there any latitude under existing law for a brand holder and a generic manufacturer to enter into an agreement which can be kept secret and not disclosed to the FTC or otherwise be made public, any latitude at all?

Mr. LEIBOWITZ. If it is a pharmaceutical patent settlement, under Hatch-Waxman, I do not believe that is possible. They must notify us under the Medicare Modernization Amendment that Senator Leahy, Senator Hatch, and this Committee passed in 2003.

Senator SPECTER. Commissioner, why not have the court which has the litigation on the underlying patent issue, litigation between the patent holder and the generic, make a decision as to whether there is an antitrust violation? We have a proliferation of cases in the Federal court. The dockets are very, very heavy. There are many illustrations where there is a public interest involved. If two private parties are involved and they come to a settlement, that is between them. But when there is a public interest involved, it is not unusual for the court to examine the public's interest and see if the public interest is being respected. Why not short-circuit all of this complex antitrust litigation by requiring the court to approve the settlement, taking into account the public interest?

Mr. LEIBOWITZ. Well, I think that is a very interesting approach, and I suppose you could—if you are interested in writing legislation to require the court to do that. Of course, we would want to work with you. But the courts have been very reluctant, as you point out, to look into the merits of the patents themselves, in part because they are interested in settlement.

Senator SPECTER. But the courts are looking into it in extraordinarily complicated cases to read these decisions in *Schering-Plough* v. *FTC* or the *Tamoxifen* case or *Valley Drugs*, you have to have a chart to diagram it to figure out all the parties. And the patent is recognized in many cases right up to the expiration date. There are very complex considerations. Why burden another court? Why not have the court making the settlement make that part of its duty? They have already got the issues before them.

Mr. LEIBOWITZ. Well, I would make a couple of points in response to that. I mean, I think it is an interesting idea, and obviously you are troubled by these settlements, as I think the whole Committee is.

First of all, it is partly the substantive standard that courts are applying. As you pointed out, the Sixth Circuit in *Cardizem* applies a sort of per se illegality approach. The *Tamoxifen* court—the Second Circuit in a 2–1 decision—and the *Schering* court apply I would almost say something that is less than rule of reason—almost sham, fraud on the Patent Office or beyond the scope of the patent in years. So I think—

Senator SPECTER. Well, wait a minute. If the court says it is rule of reason, you call it sham?

Mr. LEIBOWITZ. Well, it also says that they are looking to see whether there is a sham or fraud. In the Commission's decision in *Schering*, the FTC decision that was reversed on appeal by the Eleventh Circuit, we took a rule-of-reason approach.

Senator SPECTER. Let me interrupt you to ask you two more questions because I only have 5 minutes. When the Congress intervenes to declare conduct a per se violation of the antitrust laws, an automatic violation, we do so where we have substantial certainty as to the anticompetitive effects as to what went on. When I read these cases and you have very distinguished courts—the Eleventh Circuit on two occasions and the Second Circuit on one occasion—examining these complex factual situations—which we can't anticipate. No way we can anticipate in the law the varieties of what will come up. And they come to a conclusion that it is not anticompetitive after going through it on a detailed case-by-case analysis. Is it wise for the Congress to make a sweeping generalization to have a per se violation?

Now, the second question before my red light goes on. Once the red light goes on, you are not limited. I would like you to address, after you answer that question, what is meant by patent settlements are reasonable so long as the exclusionary effects of the settlement do not exclude the exclusionary effects of the patent?

Mr. LEIBOWITZ. The exclusionary effects of the settlement and the exclusionary effects of the patent. All right—

Senator SPECTER. Well, that is not my phraseology. That is what the courts have said.

Mr. LEIBOWITZ. Well, I think it points out how to answer your second question first—you said that you and your staffer had been trying to figure out exactly what the court was trying to say—and we have been trying to figure out the meaning of that case for quite some time ourselves. It is a very, very complicated decision, and these settlement agreements are also very complicated.

Jumping back to your first question on per se illegality, the way I read Senator Kohl's bill—I have not seen the newest iteration, but I read the bill that was introduced last year—it does not really call these deals per se illegal. It is a bright-line approach to say you can have settlements, but what you cannot do is have compensation flowing from the brand to the generic and an agreement by the generic which inherently pushes the generic toward a later entry date. And you can see, based on the chart, from 2004, before *Schering* and *Tamoxifen*, we did not see any of these deals which we would label as sort of exclusionary payments. In 2006, fiscal year 2006, after *Schering* and *Tamoxifen*, 14 out of the 28 final settlements we have looked at have resulted in what we would all call an exclusionary payment, compensation from the brand to the generic, agreement by the generic to defer entry. In terms of the first filer—and if you can lock in the first generic who files, you can often—you can pretty much—ensure subsequent generics will not be able to enter. The settlements with first filers have gone from 0 out of 8 in fiscal year 2004 before *Schering* and *Tamoxifen*, to, I think, 9 out of 11, more than 80 percent of the time.

Senator SPECTER. Well, Mr. Chairman, I am going to have to excuse myself, as I said earlier. The National Security Counselor has scheduled a meeting with Senators to talk about Iraq. But I leave this side of the podium with the distinguished Senator Hatch, who is the author of Hatch-Waxman, 1984. He is a real veteran around here, having chaired the Committee, and he knows this field backward and forwards. So I leave our side in Senator Hatch's hands.

Mr. LEIBOWITZ. Thank you, Senator Specter.

Senator HATCH. Thank you very much.

Senator KOHL. Thank you very much, Senator Specter.

Senator Hatch? Then Senator Whitehouse following you.

Senator HATCH. Thank you.

Well, Jon, welcome back to the Committee.

Mr. LEIBOWITZ. Thank you.

Senator HATCH. We are happy to have you here. We appreciate your service. In my view, the principal concern regarding settlement practices identified—

Senator KOHL. Your speaker, Orrin? Your speaker is not on.

Senator HATCH. I am sorry.

Mr. LEIBOWITZ. That is OK.

Senator HATCH. Did you hear me?

Mr. LEIBOWITZ. Yes.

Senator HATCH. OK. Other witnesses, they appear to raise two distinct sets of policy issues. Now, the first set of issues arises from the core concern that settlements predicated on an agreement in which the brand-name companies confers something of value to a generic company, a generic drug company, in exchange for a promise not to enter the market until some future date precludes the consumer benefits that would result from earlier entry by the specific generic drug company that would be a party to the litigation.

The second set of issues arises from the operation of a principle that grants the first generic company to file an ANDA, an Abbreviated New Drug Application, a 180-day period of marketing exclusivity which generally precludes the FDA from granting approval to competing generics until after the 180-day period has ended.

Mr. LEIBOWITZ. That is right, Senator. Sometimes we call that the ''bottleneck problem.''

Senator HATCH. Right. Thus, a settlement in which the generic company entitled to the exclusivity period agrees to delay its entry into the market can effectively prevent competitive entry by any other generic company. Now, while the majority of today's witnesses favor addressing one or both of these problems, there are significant differences of opinion regarding the approaches that have been proposed by members of the panel, as well as by academic experts and various Members of Congress.

Now, the principal difference voiced here today involves whether a bright-line rule prohibiting reverse payments is appropriate or whether some form of case-by-case analysis is necessary to allow litigants the flexibility to enter into settlements that potentially allow competitive entry prior to expiration of the patent at issue, which arguably provides consumer benefits that would be less certain if more cases were litigated to conclusion due to restrictions on the ability of litigants to settle prior to final judgment.

Now, it seems to me that, in addition to the options of engaging in case-by-case review of settlements or adopting a bright-line rule prohibiting reverse payments, there is a third potential approach to resolving this issue. Now, this third approach would involve removing some of the unintended consequences and perverse incentives arising from the manner in which the grant of the 180-day exclusivity period currently operates.

As nearly as I can tell, the most serious antitrust implications arise from the scenario where a settlement agreement not only prevents a single generic company from entering the market, but by virtue of the 180-day exclusivity period effectively prevents entry by any other generic competitor.

Now, a variety of suggestions have been made regarding how do you resolve or how to resolve this problem. For example, some suggest conditioning the exclusivity period on the ability of the generic company to mount a successful defense in court. This would preclude any other or any generic company that enters into a settlement from getting the benefit of the exclusivity period. Others have suggested a stronger ''use it or lose it'' provision that would ensure forfeiture of the exclusivity period if the first generic to apply for approval did not enter the market within a reasonable period of time. And, of course, the whole purpose of Hatch-Waxman was to get them into the market quickly and without having to pay practically $1 billion per drug approval that the PhRMA company has had to pay, which caused PhRMA during the negotiations on this tremendous angst, as you can imagine. They felt like—it was a very, very serious set of negotiations.

Mr. LEIBOWITZ. Sure.

Senator HATCH. Conducted in my office.

Now, Commissioner, if as many allege a significant portion of a reverse payment settlement is predicated on the ability to deter entry, then my question is whether it is sufficient to remove the ability of the parties to the settlement to obtain an exclusionary benefit from such an agreement or whether an outright prohibition of reverse payments is necessary. And I would like your opinion on that.

Mr. LEIBOWITZ. Well—

Senator HATCH. Now, let me just add one other thing.

Mr. LEIBOWITZ. Sure.

Senator HATCH. Additionally, if you would expand on your discussion of the benefits of a bright-line rule as opposed to a caseby-case analysis, I think all of us up here would appreciate it as well.

Mr. LEIBOWITZ. Well, Senator, we appreciate your concern about these exclusionary payments and the thoughtful way that you are trying to sort of look at stopping them. I read your statement from 2003 where you called some of these deals "appalling," and we want to work with you on whatever approach you want to take.

The benefits of a bright-line approach are fairly simple. First of all, you stop the problem, right? There will not be any payments from a brand—compensation flowing from a brand to a generic—and the generic deferring entry. And we have seen from 2004 to 2006 a sea change—

Senator HATCH. That also stops legitimate deals, too.

Mr. LEIBOWITZ. Well, I would not say that. We have a period of time from 2000 to 2004 where most of the industry—or the industry —believe—that all of these deals were illegal, and there were plenty of settlements during that time. I think that there were 18 in 2004 and 2005 alone before the *Schering* decision. We do not believe you would stop legitimate deals. What you would have is sort of a migration of a delayed entry date plus—from a delayed entry date plus money—to a less delayed entry date, to a different entry date, shorter, and consumers getting the benefits sooner.

The other benefit you get from the bright-line test is certainty because businesses know what they can and cannot do. And those, it seems to me, are the principal benefits of a bright-line test.

Now, I want to think a little bit about your approach and get back to you on it.

Senator HATCH. Would you?

Mr. LEIBOWITZ. It is an interesting idea, but keep in mind that there is always going to be—there may still be a huge incentive for the brands to pay the generics and the generics to stay out of the market, even if they are paying multiple generics, because of the economics of this industry. So let us get back to you on that, and we want to work with your staff.

Senator HATCH. Well, I have to admit I don't think either side would very much like that suggestion either.

Mr. LEIBOWITZ. Well, we have managed to unify the brands and generics, but only in opposition to our position on exclusion payments. So welcome to the club, Senator.

Senator HATCH. I have been there. I am in the club.

[Laugher.}

Mr. LEIBOWITZ. We are happy in our lonely eminence, though.

Senator HATCH. Thank you, Mr. Chairman.

Senator KOHL. Thank you, Senator Hatch.

Senator Whitehouse?

Senator WHITEHOUSE. Thank you, Mr. Chairman.

I had a question in response to your description of the manner in which the financial incentives of these transactions operate on the generics and on the brands, and the conclusion that they encourage anticompetitive effects and really not legitimate purposes from a consumer perspective.

To turn that on its head, can you think of any legitimate purpose for these types of pay-to-delay settlements that would cause public harm if there were to be an outright prohibition?

Mr. LEIBOWITZ. Well, again, there is a legitimate purpose to these payments. The legitimate purpose is to settle cases. But what we think in these instances in the aggregate—not necessarily with respect to each individual instance, but in the aggregate—they inherently give the patent holder, the brand, more protection than the brand ought to have. That is the problem. If you take the money or the compensation out of the equation and you make companies pick a date, an entry date based on the strength of their case—which is what happened in dozens of agreements between 2000 and early 2005—we think that consumers will be served because they will get earlier entry and cheaper drugs; drugs will go down by 20 or 30 percent with the first generic and up to 80 or 90 percent 6 months later when multiple generics come in.

We think in the aggregate the public is not served by these deals. If you take a bright-line approach—and we are, of course, willing to look at other approaches—but if you take a bright-line approach, you will encourage early generic entry, and consumers will be able to get more affordable drugs sooner rather than later. And we really do believe, as Senator Hatch alluded to, that this is really what Hatch-Waxman was all about, which has been a wonderful piece of legislation that has allowed profits for the brands and the generics, but has created a vibrant generic industry.

Senator WHITEHOUSE. Other than the public purpose of allowing cases to settle more rapidly, is there any other public purpose served by these agreements?

Mr. LEIBOWITZ. For these exclusionary agreements? No, I do not believe there is another public purpose. That is my sense, at least.

Senator WHITEHOUSE. OK. Thank you.

Mr. LEIBOWITZ. Thank you, Senator.

Senator WHITEHOUSE. Thank you, Chairman.

Senator KOHL. We thank you so much, Commissioner Leibowitz. You have added a lot to the discussion, and we appreciate your being here today.

Mr. LEIBOWITZ. Thank you so much, Senator.

[The prepared statement of Mr. Leibowitz appears as a submission for the record.]

Senator KOHL. We have a second panel, and we would like to call the four witnesses on that panel to step forward.

Our first witness is Hon. Bill Tauzin, who is President and Chief Executive Officer of PhRMA. Prior to joining PhRMA, Mr. Tauzin was a 12-term member of the U.S. House of Representatives representing Louisiana's 3rd Congressional District. Mr. Tauzin served as Chairman of the Energy and Commerce Committee from 2001 to 2004, and Mr. Tauzin graduated from Nicholls State University and earned his law degree from LSU.

Our second witness is Mr. Merril Hirsh. Mr. Hirsh is a partner at Ross, Dixon and Bell, LLP, in Washington. He has also worked as a trial attorney in the Civil Division of the U.S. Department of Justice, and he has authored several well-known articles on antitrust law.

Also joining us today is Mr. Bruce Downey, Chief Executive Officer of Barr Pharmaceuticals. Mr. Downey has received several awards for special achievements during his time in Government service, and he is Chairman of the Board of Directors for the Generic Pharmaceutical Association. Mr. Downey graduated with honors from Miami University in Ohio, and he received his law degree from Ohio State.

Finally, we will hear from Mr. Michael Wroblewski of Consumers Union, the non-profit publisher of Consumer Reports. Prior to joining Consumer Reports, Mr. Wroblewski acted as Assistant General Counsel for Policy Studies at the FTC and as attorney adviser. Mr. Wroblewski is a graduate of Loyola College and received his J.D. from the University of Texas School of Law and his MPA from the Lyndon Baines Johnson School of Public Affairs in 1992.

We hope, gentlemen, that you will limit your testimony to 5 minutes, and before you begin, I would like you to rise and take the oath of office, please. Please raise your right hand, and do you swear that the testimony you are about to give is the truth, the whole truth, and nothing but the truth, so help you God?

Mr. TAUZIN. I do.

Mr. HIRSH. I do.

Mr. DOWNEY. I do.

Mr. WROBLEWSKI. I do.

Senator KOHL. We thank you so much.

We will start with you, Mr. Wroblewski.

STATEMENT OF MICHAEL WROBLEWSKI, PROJECT DIRECTOR, CONSUMER EDUCATION AND OUTREACH, CONSUMERS UNION, THE NON-PROFIT PUBLISHER OF CONSUMER REPORTS, WASHINGTON, D.C.

Mr. WROBLEWSKI. Mr. Chairman, members of the Committee, thank you for the invitation to testify today. Consumers Union is the independent non-profit publisher of Consumer Reports. We investigate and report extensively on the issues surrounding the costs, safety, and effectiveness of prescription drugs so that we can provide our 7.3 million subscribers with expert advice to help them manage their health. Consumers Union publications carry no advertising, and we receive no commercial support.

The hearing today asks the question, "Should paying generics to prevent competition with brand drugs be prohibited?" Consumers Union responds with an emphatic "Yes." We strongly support prompt Congressional action to create a bright-line rule to end the use of patent settlements in which a brand-name company compensates a generic applicant to delay market entry. These settlements can deny consumers access to lower-priced generic drugs for many years. They also jeopardize the health of millions of Americans who have difficulty obtaining safe and effective medicines at competitive prices. I would like to highlight three reasons for our support.

First, generic drugs are critical to managing health care costs today. Health care costs continue to surge at double or triple the rate of inflation, in part due to the high cost and rate of inflation of brand-name prescription drugs. Generic drugs can dampen health inflation because they cost up to 70 or 80 percent less than the brand-name drug.

We have started a free public education initiative, "Consumer Reports Best Buy Drugs," to provide consumers with reliable, easyto-understand advice about the safest, most effective, and lowestcost prescription drug available. We currently provide information for 16 different classes of medicine, and we will expand to more classes in the future. Consumers can use this information to check to see if there is a safe, effective, and low-cost alternative to any medicine that they are taking. We encourage consumers to talk to their doctors about this information. Access to these low-cost generic drugs saves consumers substantial sums.

The second reason we support legislation is to counter the incentives that we heard about this morning that brand-name and generic companies have to enter lucrative settlement agreements. It is an economic fact that the brand company's total profits from sales of its brand drug prior to generic entry exceed the combined profits of the brand and the generic company after generic entry occurs. The upshot is that the brand-name company has a powerful incentive to pay the generic to delay entry. The payment is still less than the amount it would lose if the generic applicant entered the market.

The generic applicant, on the other hand, also gains by earning more from the settlement than it would by competing in the market. These incentives are inadvertently exacerbated by the 180-day marketing exclusivity provision of the Hatch-Waxman Act. Any settlement with the first filer blocks any subsequent generic entrants from coming into the market. So the brand-name company can forestall generic competition for years by settling with just the first-filed generic. And the generic who is first in line has powerful incentives to ask for a payment because not only will it get the payment, but it also retains its 180 days of marketing exclusivity. The irony, of course, is that the intent behind the act was to speed generic entry, not to provide the generic a windfall to delay its market entry.

The third reason we support legislation is because the courts, we believe, will not fix this in a timely manner. Two recent appellate court decisions have taken a lenient view, in our view, of these patent settlements. As a result of these rulings, a patent holder can now pay whatever it takes to buy off a generic applicant during the life of the patent. These rulings, in our view, are based on two fault premises.

First, the courts seemed to require that unless the patent can be proved to be invalid or not infringed, a court cannot declare a settlement illegal. This test, we believe, as the FTC discussed in its *Schering* opinion, may sound good in theory, but it is nearly impossible to make work from a practical point of view.

Second, these courts have elevated the generally held principle that public policy favors settlements above the statutory incentives in the act that encourage generic applicants to challenge weak patents. Industry experience shows that Congress struck the right balance when it established these statutory incentives.

Between 1992 and 2000, generic companies that challenged weak patents won their cases 73 percent of the time. Indeed, these challenges have resulted in generic entry earlier than what otherwise would have occurred absent the generic challenge.

For all three of these reasons, we urge Congress to act now so that consumers get the benefit of timely generic competition.

Thank you very much, and I would be happy to take any questions that you have now or at the end of the panel.

[The prepared statement of Mr. Wroblewski appears as a submission for the record.]

Senator KOHL. Thank you, Mr. Wroblewski. We will first hear testimony from Mr. Tauzin and then Mr. Hirsh and then Mr. Downey.

STATEMENT OF BILLY TAUZIN, PRESIDENT AND CHIEF EXECUTIVE OFFICER, PHARMACEUTICAL RESEARCH AND MANUFACTURERS OF AMERICA (PHRMA), WASHINGTON, D.C.

Mr. TAUZIN. Senator Kohl, thank you. This is my first opportunity to testify before Congress, and I welcome the chance to be before your Committee. Senator Hatch, Senator Whitehouse, I also thank you for the chance.

Let me first acknowledge something. I am not only the President of PhRMA; I also a cancer survivor, like Senator Specter. Just 2 years ago, I finished chemotherapy following a cancer that left me with about a 5-percent chance of survival. And yet, after that year of chemotherapy, with a brand-new miracle drug that came out of this industry, I am with you today and with my family, and I have them to thank for that.

And so, like Senator Specter, I am deeply concerned not only from my position as a representative of this industry but also as a patient who is still next week going through another cancer test, as I have to go through it every 4 months.

I am interested in making sure that the process by which these new miracle drugs are brought to market is not severely damaged by changes in public policy, that we take very careful concern for the patent protection that is provided, the incentive to spend the $50 billion that was spent last year in trying to find a new cancer drugs that saves lives today.

So let me start by doing what Senator Specter did in his opening statement, which is to illustrate that this is about a 14.2-year process. When a company that is inventing a new drug that is going to save our lives or battle disease for us first files for its patent and it gets its patent approved, it needs another 14.2 years of that patent life just to bring it to market, to do all the testing, the clinical analysis, the proof to the FDA, the proof to itself that it has a product that is both efficacious and also worth the risk, because every drug, every medicine, has certain risks attached to it, certain side effects. It has got to make sure before it brings it to market that it is safe and effective, in effect. So it uses about 14 years of its patent life and spending about $1 billion to bring that drug to market so that my life could be saved 2 years ago.

That is the story. But that is not the end of the story. The next chart shows you what happens next in comparison to other products that are invented in our society. What happens next is that after the final market approval, there is only about 5 or 6 years left, generally, on the patent life of a brand-new drug, a cancerfighting drug. And if you get the benefit of patent term restoration that comes from Hatch-Waxman, the maximum ever you can have on your patent life is about 14 years. The average today is 11 to 12 years.

Now, I am going to ask one of my colleagues to pass out a pen to you. It is a little cheap pen. It does not violate your rules so you can keep it as a gift. There are some words on it. It says, ''This pen's patents have more protection than those for cancer medicine.'' And I am going to illustrate to you how true that is.

By the way, unfortunately, this pen is made in Mexico, like so many products that we buy in America. But it was patented here in this country.

I am going to prove it to you. This pen and other products we manufacture, invent and manufacture in this country, go through the same patent approval process as a drug, except they do not have to go through 14 years of testing to see whether they are safe and effective. They go to market immediately. So the guy who invents this pen starts selling it the day after he gets his patent approved, protected by the patent. The drug, on the other hand, has to spend about 14 years in testing. And so the effective protection for this pen is about $17_{1.2}$ years. The protection for the patent on a new medicine that saves my life and saves yours is about 11 to 12 years.

Now, the settlements we are talking about, Senator Kohl, involve challenges to those patents. Hatch-Waxman allows that challenge to come as early as 4 years after the drug goes to market. It involves a challenge to the patent. It involves somebody saying, ''Your patent is invalid. You did not do it right.'' It involves somebody saying, you know, ''We are going to copy your work, copy your drug, and put it on the market as a generic product because we think our drug does not infringe on your patent,'' or, ''Your patent is invalid.'' Start with that proposition. It is a challenge to the patent, and a desire to enter the marketplace before you would ordinarily be entitled to enter the marketplace.

Now, Hatch-Waxman encourages that, and before Hatch-Waxman, about 20 percent of the drugs sold in America were generic drugs. Today 60 percent are generic drugs, according to the latest numbers. The utility and usefulness of generic drugs in America exceeds that of any country in the world. Generic drugs are very important to the marketplace of health care in this country. We can see that. We admit that. We support that.

What we are asking today is, however, to think very carefully about whether or not you interfere with, in a broad and overreaching way, the ability of generic drugs and patent drugs to settle these kind of cases that challenge the validity of patents.

Now, why do we ask you to be careful? One, I am not here to defend bad or ugly settlements that do not meet a test of antitrust law. They ought to be discarded, and the FTC has that authority today to invalidate any of those settlements. Every settlement has to be turned over to the FTC and the Justice Department. Somebody gets a second look at it, and they can say, ''No, sorry. That settlement violates antitrust law. We turn it down.'' The FTC does that. It is hard work. They do not like to do it. I understand that.

Sometimes the courts will overturn them, as they did in *Schering-Plough*. Sometimes the courts will agree with them. But this Congress several years ago declared that any one of these settlements have to go through that test. If you want to put them through a different test, fine. But to outlaw them completely does something I hope we don't do for the sake of consumers, not just for drugs companies, but for patients like me. What those settlements very often do is bring generic drugs sooner to the marketplace than they would be allowed to if those patents were respected until the end of their patent term.

What very often a good settlement does is end costly litigation that consumers pay for in the end and end uncertainty in the marketplace, which is critical for this model to work, and allow generic drugs on the marketplace sooner than later.

Now, you heard a number saying, well, the companies lose 73 percent of the cases. That is not true. Seventy-three percent of the cases represents the times the company lost, including the times the company settled. If you look at current rates, you will see that companies are winning more cases than losing them now. And the reason they are winning them more is they are learning from their past mistakes. They are learning how to write better patents and defend them more properly.

So if you don't allow settlements, if you don't allow the good settlements that are in the interest of the consumer to go forward, the ones the FTC would approve, the ones the Justice Department would approve, you may have the reverse effect of hurting consumers by denying them the chance to get a generic into the marketplace even during a valid patent term. That is what settlements do.

So here I am at the Clint Eastwood moment. Clint Eastwood made some great films. One I love is ''The Good, The Bad and the Ugly.'' Now, he was like you. He was a law keeper—a law maker and a law keeper and a law enforcer. And he rode into town, and his job was to kill the bad and the ugly, but to protect the good. And so I ask you one thing on behalf of patients like me and all of us who depend upon this process to keep these miracle drugs flowing, and there are 2,000 more in the pipeline right now, 600 new cancer medicines in the pipeline right now. If we are going to keep this model working and new cancer drugs patented and approved and the new drugs for diabetes and heart failure and everything else, I ask you please not to shoot the good while you are trying to kill the bad and the ugly.

The process ought to pick the bad settlements out and kill them. It ought to pick the bad and the ugly and say you cannot go forward. But you ought not sweep away the good settlements that end unnecessary litigation that is very expensive. Some expert testified 27 cents of every dollar spent in research and development is spent in court fighting over this stuff instead. You ought not throw out the good settlements that work to bring generics sooner to the marketplace than later because it ends the disputes, ends the litigation, ends the payment to lawyers, and instead flows these products to patients who need them.

Don't shoot the good. Let's just keep shooting the bad and the ugly.

Thank you, sir.

[The prepared statement of Mr. Tauzin appears as a submission for the record.]

Senator KOHL. Thank you, Mr. Tauzin.

Mr. Hirsh?

STATEMENT OF MERRIL HIRSH, PARTNER, ROSS, DIXON AND BELL, LLP, WASHINGTON, D.C.

Mr. HIRSH. Thank you, Senator. I want to thank the Committee and its staff for affording me the opportunity to comment on the proposed Preserve Access to Generics Act. Although on this issue my law firm has generally represented the interests of companies who pay the cost of drugs through self-insurance, the views I express today are my own and not necessarily those of either my firm or any of its clients. In fact, my firm represents both plaintiffs and defendants in various types of litigation, and I hope that whatever thoughts I can convey to the Committee reflect the experience of having been on both sides.

On March 20, 2006, the Philadelphia Business Journal reported on an interview with the chief executive officer of Cephalon, Incorporated. Cephalon had settled patent challenges to Provigil, a drug for sleep disorders, by paying a total of at least $136 million to several of its generic competitors. By settling, Cephalon avoided a ruling on the generics' arguments that Cephalon's patent was invalid and that the patent was not infringed in any event by the generic substitutes.

As the CEO explained to analysts about the settlement, ''A lot of [Wall Street's enthusiasm for Cephalon's stock] is a result of patent litigation getting resolved for Provigil. We were able to get six more years of patent protection. That's $4 billion in sales that no one expected.''

Now, you would ordinarily think that paying off a competitor to obtain 6 more years of patent protection and $4 billion more in sales than you expected would be viewed as anticompetitive, and there is currently a lawsuit pending arguing that this violates the antitrust laws. The defendants in that case, however, have moved to dismiss it. They are arguing that, even when the CEO admits that the payments achieve patent protection no one expected, these payments cannot, as a matter of law, violate the current antitrust laws.

I think defendants should lose that motion, but honestly, illogical as the motion seems, it is not frivolous, given the current state of the law. The plaintiffs in the *Tamoxifen* case have petitioned the Supreme Court for a review of the Second Circuit's decision that people have discussed here that otherwise may effectively immunize brand and generic companies from paying any amount of money to resolve any patent case that was not a sham case to begin with. And, as the FTC has reported and Commissioner Leibowitz discussed today, a recent spate of reverse payment settlements shows companies clearly emboldened to make these settlements unless and until they are told not to. These reverse payment settlements are indeed anticompetitive, and they defeat the purposes of the Hatch-Waxman Act.

Now, I think it is impossible not to be moved by Representative Tauzin's personal story and his basic point of attempting to capture the good and only deal with the bad and the ugly. The problem is that reverse payment settlements are the bad in this case, and, in fact, the preservation of reverse payment settlements doesn't preserve the type of protections he is talking about to the patents.

What reverse payment settlements do is create a tremendous incentive to do two things: first, to have generic companines pick patent fights in the hopes of being able to be paid off for dropping them; and, second, to settle those fights in ways that do no justice to the Hatch-Waxman Act and provide no benefits to consumers.

Brand companies are not made better off by a system that encourages people to sue them without the risk of putting drugs onto market in the hopes of being paid off with enormous amounts of money available to pay them. That does not lead to fewer lawsuits. It leads to more lawsuits. And more lawsuits are not better. In fact, not having lawsuits in the first place is better than settling lawsuits after they are brought.

Second, once lawsuits are brought, reverse payment settlements are not the only way to settle them. They are a convenient way to settle them. They are convenient because there is an extraordinary incentive, as everyone has discussed today. A delay for some of these drugs involves a million dollars a day—a million dollars a day for each day the generic entry is excluded, a million dollars in additional sales. There is an enormous incentive for companies who legitimately are interested in profit for their shareholders to engage in a sharing of this money rather than a result that actually brings down the cost for consumers.

If you eliminate the reverse payment settlements, and this is the reason you need a bright-line rule to solve this problem, you eliminate that possibility. You allow for lawsuits being brought where there are genuine patent challenges. This is where the generic genuinely intends to market the product and not just hold up the brand company. The brand and generic companies are forced to negotiate at arm's-length over when the generic can come in, and their agreement harnesses the market force of an arm's-length negotiation, not just to benefit the parties involved, but to benefit consumers.

Courts are unable to deal with this problem because it involves a policy judgment that is Congress' to make. That is why I strongly support the legislation before the Committee.

Thank you, Senator.

[The prepared statement of Mr. Hirsh appears as a submission for the record.]

Senator KOHL. Thank you, Mr. Hirsh.

Mr. Downey?

STATEMENT OF BRUCE L. DOWNEY, CHAIRMAN AND CHIEF EXECUTIVE OFFICER, BARR PHARMACEUTICALS, INC., WASHINGTON, D.C.

Mr. DOWNEY. Thank you, Senator. It is very nice to be here today appearing before the Senate Judiciary Committee again. I am the Chairman and Chief Executive Officer of Barr Pharmaceuticals, one of the largest generic companies in the country. We are also probably the most prolific challenger of brand patents. In my tenure at Barr, we have brought over 30 cases challenging the patents protecting pharmaceutical products. We have completed about half of those cases; about half are still pending. Of those we completed, 14 were settled, and 13 of those settlements brought products to market prior to patent expiry—that is, that shortened patent life of the brand product allowed us to get into the market and compete earlier than we otherwise could.

Now, we have also taken some cases to trial, and I think in the statements of the Senators and the testimony of my colleagues, two of our cases have been prominently mentioned. One is the Prozac case, and it has been the poster child of what should happen; that is, you should take a case to trial, win it, and bring a product to market. The second was our *Tamoxifen* case. It has been the poster child for what is wrong. You should not settle a case in exchange for consideration other than early entry. I want to examine those two cases in detail because both of those cases brought significant value to consumers, and both of those settlements would have been impossible if this legislation were to pass. Let me start with the Prozac case because I think that is the most misunderstood.

We brought the case against the Prozac patent. There were three claims: one, it was invalid for double patenting; two, it was invalid because of the best mode rule; and, third, it was invalid because of the inequitable conduct of the Lilly Company at the Patent Office. We lost the double patenting and best mode arguments in summary judgment before the district court. We thought those were our best claims. The judge dismissed them, and we were stuck now with our inequitable conduct claim, which we thought was the weakest. The judge set it down for trial. To take that case to trial on appeal would have taken an additional year before we could get our other claims before the court of appeals. And we settled that claim on the eve of trial for a cash payment, which would have been prohibited by this legislation. But taking that payment, settling that claim, allowed us to appeal the best mode and double patenting claim to the court of appeals, which we ultimately won. It shortened the case by a year, allowed us to bring generic Prozac to market a year earlier than we could if we had gone to trial on inequitable conduct. And that reverse payment saved consumers about a billion and a half dollars. So in that case, the reverse payment actually had the exact effect that all of the other witnesses supporting the legislation want it to have.

Now, in *Tamoxifen*, we tried the case and we won, and our opponents appealed. All of our strong arguments, in my opinion, we lost at trial, and we had one argument remaining for the court of appeals, and that was the inequitable conduct case. We settled that on appeal because we thought we were going to lose. We took payment, we took a license, and we entered the market early with *Tamoxifen*. And over the course of our license, we saved consumers about $300 million on that product.

Now, this was a great laboratory experiment because, following our case where we accepted this payment, which others think is illegal, three other generic companies tried to challenge that patent. All three of them went to trial. All three of them lost. All three of them went to the court of appeals, and all three of them lost. I believe had we not settled the case and entered the product with our license from Zeneca, we also would have lost and consumers would have been harmed.

So those two cases where we accepted what are called reverse payments saved consumers nearly $2 billion that otherwise would have been impossible. So I think the legislation will have very serious unintended consequences. It will reduce the number of patent cases we bring. It will force us to take each of the cases that are brought to trial and sort of fight to the death. And then, finally, it will prohibit settlements that shorten the patent life and bring products to market sooner than we otherwise could.

You know, it is not really the reverse payment that keeps products off the market. It is the patent. The patent is a monopoly granted by the Government that is entitled to a presumption of validity. It can only be overturned by a showing of clear and convincing evidence. You know, we do not bring products to market in the face of a patent because of the damages we risk. And I also disagree with the success rate that has been given here. It is not 70 percent. Our success rate in cases that have gone to trial is like 40 percent, and that is in part because we have reached reasoned settlements that shorten the patent life, we get less than we would get if we win, we get more than we would get if we lose, and that benefit is transferred to consumers. They get more than they would get if we lose the case; they get less than if we would win it. I think that is the way all settlements are. They are a compromise. Each side gets something. In this case, we compromised on the length of the patent term. We shortened the patent life. We were in earlier. Other people can challenge the patent if they want.

Now, there is an anomaly, Senator Hatch, and I will point to that in the 180-day exclusionary provision. The MMA of 2004 does have sort of a loophole that makes it hard for second challengers to challenge the patent, and I would like to work with the Committee to help solve that problem. But it is not solved by the proposed legislation. The proposed legislation deals with settlements and not with the bottleneck loophole.

I would be happy to take any questions that you have.

[The prepared statement of Mr. Downey appears as a submission for the record.]

Senator KOHL. Thank you.

A questions for Mr. Tauzin. Your organization, as we all know, represents many large pharmaceutical companies. Isn't it just common sense, Mr. Tauzin, that if a brand-name drug company can forestall competition by paying a generic company some fraction of its profits on a drug that it will do so?

Mr. TAUZIN. Not necessarily. Again, remember, Senator Kohl, this is a patent dispute fight. If it has a great patent and that patent language has been tested and fought out in court before and proven to be valid, it has great incentive to go ahead and say, ''No, I am sorry. We are not going to settle with you. We are going to defend our patent all the way, and we are going to prevail because we have got a great patent.''

Now, if there is any kind of question about it, the incentives flow in both directions. I think you have heard the arguments from the generic association about why they have an incentive to settle on some cases, where they think they might have a chance of losing, and yet they can get their generic drug to market a little quicker if they settle.

In the case of the patent company, if they think there is some doubt about winning the case, they do what all lawyers do when fighting a case. You figure out whether your risk of losing merits the risk of settlement. In that case, very often in that discussion a settlement is reached where a generic does come into the market, even in the face of what otherwise they believe is a valid patent.

But the incentives flow in both directions, and they are going to be different in every case. And in some cases, as you pointed out, as Mr. Leibowitz pointed out, those settlements need to be examined to see whether or not they reach a public interest standard. I agree with that.

But the bottom line is that the incentives work in both directions, and in some cases, in some 50-some-odd percent of the cases lately, the patent companies go all the way to trial because they believe they have a valid patent and they have a right to depend upon it.

Mr. Leibowitz, by the way, is not against patents, I do not believe. I do not believe he is against patent protection. Neither is this Committee. He worked for the Motion Picture Association and got a 95-year patent on Mickey Mouse. You know, on the other hand, a drug that saved my life and others' lives may get only 11 or 12 years of protection. That is our concern. If you mess with that model too much, you begin damaging the incentive to go out and spend the billion to invest in new medicine. That is happening all over the world. That is why 70 percent of the new medicines invented in the world are invented here in America, because we still, to the extent we can, give some reward for somebody spending those billions of dollars to invent those new medicines.

So all we ask is that whatever you do in this area—and we will work with you to try to find a solution that makes sense for everyone here—is that we do not end up throwing out the good with the bad.

Senator KOHL. Mr. Downey, the FTC reports that in the year after the two court decisions that we have covered here today, allowing these reverse payment settlements, half of all patent settlements contained terms in which the brand-name company paid generic in return for the generic's agreement in keeping the drug off the market. And as we have discussed, in the year before that court decision, no patent settlements contained any such terms. So doesn't this data indicate that going forward, unless we do something about that by way of our legislation, increasingly there are going to be financial settlements arrived at?

Mr. DOWNEY. Well, I do not believe the data is exactly right. First, I would say the later settlements where there were payments, it is not the payment that keeps the product off the market. It is the patent. And in one of those cases—it happens to be ours I know about—there was a compromise where we entered the market years before patent expiry, but some number of years in the future, there was 12, 15 years left on the patent, and we compromised at a point sort of halfway in between.

In addition to that, we had some other arrangement with the brand company. We think that is very pro-competitive—pro-competitive in two parts: one, because we shortened the patent life; and, two, because we got this collateral benefit in the other part of the deal—all of which was submitted to the FTC, and if they think it is improper, they could challenge it. I think they would lose, but that data has been made available as a requirement under existing law.

Also, I disagree that the years before those cases there were not settlements that involved other consideration, because I know we had at least one.

Senator KOHL. Mr. Wroblewski, would you like to comment on this question? Then Mr. Hirsh.

Mr. WROBLEWSKI. The only thing I would like to add is the statistic rate that I quoted in my testimony in terms of how frequently the generic challenger wins, that statistic comes from looking at all of the court cases—not including the settlements—but just the court cases. Between 1992 and 2000, there were 30 decisions of a court, and in 22 of those instances, the generic won. So that is the 73 percent. That study ended in 2000, 2001, and that has not yet been updated.

I am familiar with a study by the American Intellectual Property Law Committee that has basically come up with the same 70-percent number by looking at the defendant winning in patent litigations, the challenger basically, in a broader spectrum of industries, and it has been right around 70 percent.

So I think I will stick with, you know, that the incentive has provided —has not been misused to challenge patents, as they are picking the right patents to challenge.

Mr. TAUZIN. Senator, if I could jump in, we are using data from 2004 to 2006. That is much later than this study which did not include settlements. And the data between 2004 to 2006 indicates innovative companies prevailed at the appellate level 52 percent of the time.

Senator KOHL. All right. Mr. Hirsh, do you want to make a comment?

Mr. HIRSH. Yes. I think where the disconnect is going on in this discussion is as follows: As a lawyer handling commercial cases and intellectual property cases, you are frequently faced with the situation where one of the possible outcomes you can negotiate is anticompetitive. Negotiations inherently look for win-wins between parties because there are ways of narrowing gaps between people who would otherwise disagree. And I don't know any commercial litigator who has not been in some situation where at some point you look at someone across a table and you say, ''Well, we could do that, but we can't because it violates the antitrust laws. We need to find another solution.''

What happens in those circumstances is not that the case does not settle. What happens in those situations is it settles in a way that is lawful.

In a Hatch-Waxman settlement, the question is what is the money part being paid for. As Commissioner Leibowitz talked about the question, nobody is against having cases brought that are legitimate. Nobody is against having brand companies defend patents to the end if they think they are right, or both parties bringing them to litigation and getting a litigated result if they think they are right, or settling those cases.

If they settle the case on the basis that they cannot exchange money, the terms of the negotiation is over when can the generic enter the market, with the generic incentivized to enter the market sooner. The sooner the generic can enter into the market, the sooner the generic can share in some of the profits that come from the drug.

If there is money that changes hands in addition to that, what is the brand company paying the generic the money for? It is understandable that the brand is willing to pay it. It is understandable that the generic is happy to take it. But the logical terms of the negotiation is that the brand is paying the benefit of having less competition, of moving the entry date back.

Now, it is quite correct, as Mr. Downey points out, you have settlements that have components of both: there is a payment, and the generic can come in before the end of the patent. There are situations in which the generic may not feel that they have a 100-percent winning case and they would rather settle.

The problem with the reverse payment is what you are paying for is to have that settlement have the effect of having the generic come in later. That is what the money is being exchanged hands for, and that is what is anticompetitive. If you eliminate that incentive, the case will still settle if the parties think they are weak, and the case will not settle if the parties think their cases are strong. What will happen is that the settlement will reflect the strength of the patent instead of ignoring that. That is why it is better.

Senator KOHL. Thank you. Before we—I am sorry. Mr. Tauzin, go ahead.

Mr. TAUZIN. Can I just add one thing? There is a great dispute as to whether or not, when you eliminate the exchange of things of value, you are going to encourage or discourage settlements. I can tell you in the *Schering-Plough* case, for example, there was a licensing agreement that went along with the settlement. If you could not do that licensing agreement, our information is that settlement probably would not have gone forward. That is the one the FTC disapproved of and the court approved of. That is a case where the settlement did bring the generic product into the marketplace sooner.

You are going to get a dispute over that, and you will always have that. That is our point, that case-by-case when you look at them, you are going to see some cases where a settlement made sense for the consumer and another case where it possibly did not, where you ought to say, sorry, that cannot go forward. That is a different matter.

Senator KOHL. Last comment, Mr. Downey.

Mr. DOWNEY. Yes, a very important point here. The collateral agreements that narrow the gap are not always cash payments. In fact, they rarely are in our case. They involve some other asset that has a different value for us than it does the brand. Sometimes, for example, we have purchased a product from the brand at a price we think is favorable—it is an asset that is not key to them—as part of the settlement where we have shortened the patent life. In other cases, we have licensed a patent from a brand as part of a settlement where we have shortened the patent life. In other cases, we have agreed to co-promote products for the brand company as part of the settlement where we have shortened the patent life. In other cases, we have entered into an R&D agreement with a brand company as part of a settlement where we shortened the patent life.

So these collateral agreements provide value to us, value to the brand, and simultaneously allow us to shorten the patent life. And the reason they are very important is the parties cannot always agree, in fact, seldom agree on the probability of success. And so you have some rough approximation—we might think it is 50 percent, they might think they are going to win 70 percent of the time—and you bridge that gap through these agreements that provide value to both us and to the brand company and ultimately to the consumer as these things work their way through the system.

It is very important that these other opportunities be allowed, or the settlements really are not going to happen. That is why I think the law as it is drafted would take every case to trial, every case to appeal, and there would be very, very few settlements.

Senator KOHL. Very good. Before we turn to Senator Hatch, Senator Schumer has requested a minute or two to make some comments before he has to leave.

STATEMENT OF HON. CHARLES E. SCHUMER, A U.S. SENATOR FROM THE STATE OF NEW YORK

Senator SCHUMER. Thank you, Mr. Chairman. I apologize. Finance is voting on the minimum wage, and they do not allow proxy voting. That is the only Committee I am on that does not allow proxy voting, so I apologize and thank you both for your indulgence. And thank you for having the hearing today.

As you know, Mr. Chairman, I asked the Committee to hold a hearing on this issue last May, and I am very pleased that you in always your wisdom have chosen it as one of the first hearings in the new 110th Congress. Many of us in this room are strong proponents of competition that leads to lower drug prices for consumers, most notably my friend Senator Hatch, who paved the way in 1984 with the bipartisan Hatch-Waxman Act. And in 2003, I authored with Senator McCain a law that closed loopholes that had gradually been opened up since Hatch-Waxman was passed in 1984. I worked closely, as Mr. Barr knows, with the generic drug industry to try and close those loopholes. They helped restore the integrity of Hatch-Waxman and preserved access of consumers to generic drugs.

But it seems that every time we close a door on ways to game the system, PhRMA opens up a window, and I really regret to say that in this one, they are joined by many of my friends in the generic drug industry.

Hatch-Waxman was written to help consumers, to lower the price of drugs for everyday people, not to pad profits for company shareholders. When the law is allowed to function properly, consumers win, $8 to $10 billion a year worth. But time and time again, we have needed to amend this law because the industry, instead of spending its time innovating new drugs, comes up with new ways to exploit loopholes and increases its profit share at the expense of consumers. Usually, these loopholes pit brand drug companies against generics, but this time they are actually working together to leave consumers out in the cold. So now we are seeing instances where some brand drug companies are working with some generic drug companies to make anticompetitive deals that benefit everyone except the consumer. Give money to the generic company to go away so that the brand company can continue to enjoy a monopoly on the market. And, you know,

I do not entirely blame the generic drug company. Being sued is no fun. Any company threatened with or actually faced with a lawsuit has good reason to find a quick way out. And these companies, face the facts, even though they do a lot of good and bring the cost of drugs down, are not public servants. You are supposed to serve your shareholders. And so if the company sees an opportunity, the generic company, to increase their profits, they are legally bound to do so. But we are not, and that is where the Government comes in, because we are the only player in this game who has the power to protect the consumer, preserve competition, and restore the playing field to its original condition.

There is simply no reason to allow these anticonsumer settlements. Companies only utilize them when the opportunity exists, and otherwise they function as the Hatch-Waxman law had intended. For 5 out of the last 7 years, it has been illegal for generic companies to accept money, as Mr. Downey noted, in exchange for staying out of the market. Yet competition did not drop off. In fact, the number of patent challenges actually increased during the time these particular settlements were outlawed, from 35 challenges in 2001 to 97 in 2004. It was not until two courts suddenly legalized these payoffs in 2005 that all of a sudden the industry cannot survive without them. And let me reiterate: The Leahy-Kohl-Grassley-Schumer bill will not prohibit drug companies from reaching settlements. It only prohibits settlements in which a brand company pays a generic company to stay off the market, something that generic companies in every other instance fight tooth and nail. They want to get into the market. And here all of a sudden they are saying, Oh, no, give us some money and we will stay away. And who is hurt? The consumer.

So there is no reason to make these specific settlements illegal. We just need to make sure that the bright line we all keep talking about is the right line and that we do not accidentally trap settlements that are pro-consumer in with the bad ones. When consumers have access to lower-cost drugs, we all win. But as long as we let stand the appellate court decisions that encourage brand and generic companies to split up the pie between them and not give the consumer even a forkful, we are accepting higher drug prices for the average American.

Mr. Chairman, I am proud to have worked with you and your very capable staff over the last several months on this issue and proud to be a cosponsor of the act. I look forward to continue to working with you to prohibit settlements that harm the consumer, and I would ask unanimous consent, because now they are beeping me and I have got to go to vote, to submit written questions for the record.

Thank you, Mr. Chairman. Thank you, Senator Hatch.

Senator KOHL. Senator Hatch?

STATEMENT OF HON. ORRIN G. HATCH, A U.S. SENATOR FROM THE STATEMENT OF UTAH

Senator HATCH. Well, Hatch-Waxman was not written just for consumers. It was written for consumers. It was written to create the modern generic drug industry, which it did. Like you say, it went from about 16 percent to now close to 60 percent.

It was written to provide some of the solutions that Mr. Tauzin mentioned of loss of patent life that just was not fair. If you create a widget or a pen, you have got 20 years of patent life. Like you say, 17$_{1.2}$ years and you can have market exclusivity for that pen that you used here today. Drug companies are spending up to \$1 billion for every drug they create and lose up to 15 years of patent life, leaving them 5 years left in some cases. So we did a classic compromise by—and the bill is called the Drug Price Competition Patent Term Restoration bill.'' And because of that, PhRMA has done very well. Generics have become dominant in the drug field without killing PhRMA, and consumers have benefited greatly.

Now, what we are concerned about here is there are some things that are wrong with the way this works, and Mr. Wroblewski and Mr. Hirsh raise some issues here. And so do Mr. Tauzin and Mr. Downey. Now, interestingly enough, I know—I believe I know all four of you, but I specifically know Mr. Downey and Mr. Tauzin very well. Mr. Tauzin and I sat for hours and hours month after month on that Medicare Modernization Act, and I saw a real master in action there trying to bring about a way whereby consumers would benefit, which they certainly have.

Mr. Downey has been one of the leaders, and he took a company that was not all that dominant to where it is not only dominant in the generic drug industry, but also becoming very influential in the area of the PhRMA industry as well. And I commend you for that.

But, you know, let's be honest about it. This I don't think should be a question between a bright line and doing nothing. There may be some way that we can do this so that consumers benefit, generics benefit, brand-name companies benefit. If we take the incentives away, which the House bill just did a week ago—we are the leading pharmaceutical country in the world because we have— even with the fact that we lose so many years of patent life, because of a robust set of PhRMA companies and set of generic companies.

Well, my principal question for the panel is the same, and I will start with you, Mr. Tauzin, and I for one know both of you have benefited from very important drug discoveries. And thank God for that. You are both tremendous people, leading your industries in what I consider to be tremendously influential ways. And I believe that you two consumer advocates are doing the same for your people.

But my principal question for the panel is the same one that I focused on with Commissioner Leibowitz. I would like each of you to expand on the arguments regarding the relative merits of a bright-line rule versus a case-by-case review— you will notice I did not say do nothing, but a case-by-case review—and then I would like each of you to address the question of whether it would be sufficient to reduce the incentives to enter into settlements predicated on reverse payments by modifying the 180-day exclusivity period.

Now, it seems to me that changing the way the exclusivity period operates would substantially reduce the incentives to agree to reverse payments agreements, or whether you believe adopting a bright-line rule—and I take it the two in the middle probably do agree with that—whether that bright-line rule is necessary.

I would also be interested in hearing specific changes to the 180-day exclusivity period that you would support.

Why don't we start with you, Mr. Downey, and then go across the table. And then I have a couple of questions for Mr. Downey, if I could, before this is over.

Mr. Downey. Well, as I have testified, we oppose the bright-line rule. We think it has very serious unintended consequences that are negative for our company, for our industry, and for consumers, and I—

Senator Hatch. Well, you have argued that the bill would prohibit several of the statements which occurred over the past decade, even those which have allowed generics to enter the market earlier than would have been possible had the lawsuit not been brought or lost.

Mr. Downey. It probably would have prohibited half a dozen or more of the settlements that we have that brought the products to market earlier than patent—

Senator Hatch. Would you provide the Committee with the cost to consumers if this legislation had been in effect in the last 10 years, this proposed legislation?

Mr. Downey. Yes, we can provide that, and I have said just in the two cases—

Senator Hatch. Could you do that for us?

Mr. Downey. The two instances I testified about, *Prozac* and *Tamoxifen*, those two alone saved consumers over a billion and a half dollars, and clearly would not have been available had we not settled.

Senator Hatch. Almost $2 billion, actually.

Mr. DOWNEY. Well, *Prozac* was decided a year early. We would have still gotten some benefit in *Prozac*, but the year accelerated would have been lost without the settlement.

Senator HATCH. OK.

Mr. DOWNEY. Now, I also heard from Senator Specter what I thought was a very interesting idea in the case-by-case method, and that is to have the settlements presented to the court for approval at the time they are entered into. That is something that is very standard procedure in securities litigation and class action litigation to ensure that members of the class are adequately protected by the settlement. And I think it would be entirely appropriate to have those settlements presented to the court for the court's review. I think that would be an excellent suggestion or alternative to the proposed legislation.

Senator HATCH. The court could decide at that time whether it was a violation—

Mr. DOWNEY. Yes, they could decide at the time whether it was a violation or not. You know, without taking too much time, I think there is a very clear area of the law—and this applies to patents all over, you know, whether it is electronics, automotives, plastics, whatever—and that is, patent holders have a monopoly that is granted by the Government, and they can settle cases so long as they do not expand that monopoly power that has already been granted; that is, they cannot expand its scope or the duration of the patent.

If you take the *Andrx* case, the Sixth Circuit case, which ruled that something was per se legal, that case did expand the patent, and it was properly found to be unlawful under existing law. The *Tamoxifen* case and the *Valley Drug* case did not expand the scope of the patent and properly determined under existing law to be valid, and I think that kind of analysis could be handled by the court very readily and under existing law and then there is no need for legislation.

Senator HATCH. Before I move across the table, let me just say while you are talking, why can't the money that is now paid as a pharmaceutical patent settlement—or pharmaceutical patent settlements, why can't that money always be translated into additional days of early market entry for the generic company?

Mr. DOWNEY. Because the parties generally have a different view of the case in two different respects: one, the strength of the case; and, second, the value of the entry for the generic and the cost of allowing that entry from the brand. And those variables change over time, as you learn more about the case or as new products get introduced or whatever. So there is a huge amount of uncertainty. Just restricting it to that one variable of early entry, I think it is very hard to bridge the gap on these variables. We have had settlement discussions in 20- some cases that I have conducted and settled about three-quarters of them. And when we cannot settle, it is because you cannot bridge that gap.

What these collateral arrangements do, whether it is an R&D partnership, whether it is buying a product, licensing a patent, these other exchanges of value have different—those assets have different value for the two parties, and you are able to bridge the gap that you cannot bridge on the early entry through these collateral agreements. In every case that we have settled, except *Prozac*, we got early entry, and that reduced the patent life, demonstrably pro-competitive, and many of the settlements had these other collateral issues. The only ones that get settled for early entry only are two kinds of cases: one, where the product itself is very small, or where the remaining patent life is very short. In those two cases, we have settled maybe a half a dozen times for early entry only without some collateral agreement. The rest of the time the complexity that I have just described makes it impossible to bridge the gap on early entry alone, and it is most readily bridged by these collateral agreements, which we have done a number of.

Senator HATCH. All right. Thank you.

Mr. Wroblewski?

Mr. WROBLEWSKI. Three thoughts to relate to you.

First, in terms of why we support the bright-line rule, other than what we talked about in the testimony, in the written testimony, when you go back and you look at really the only comprehensive study of agreements in which each agreement has been examined, settlement agreement, which is in the FTC's Generic Drug Study, from the period 1992 through 2002 every settlement agreement that had some type of compensation being paid from the brand company to the generic company, in nearly every one of them the entry date was actually at the date when the patent expired. There may be anecdotal evidence in terms of maybe entry comes in 6 months before the patent expires. But if you look at the evidence—and the only evidence that is really out there in terms of an examination of each agreement—my concern is that in the future they will just push the generic entry basically in line with when the patent expires. That, of course, goes against the entire intent in my reading of Hatch-Waxman.

Senator HATCH. But if the court had a right to review that, I think the court would find that offensive.

Mr. WROBLEWSKI. Sure. My only concern with having a court review it is, unlike the idea of when, say in an antitrust case, the judge is looking to see whether the class action settlement is fair, it is really applying the same law that it has just had the trial on. In this particular instance, you are asking a patent judge who has just been looking at the patent issues to now apply a whole different —a new set of laws. They are going to have to look at antitrust law to measure whether the settlement is in the public interest. And my concern with that is, with the split in circuits between the Sixth Circuit and the Second Circuit, which law, what law is the patent judge now going to apply when looking at the settlement agreement from an antitrust point of view?

My concern with using kind of a case-by-case analysis is that my reading of *Tamoxifen* and the *Schering* decision, the Eleventh Circuit's *Schering* decision, I do not really believe that the courts have given sufficient deference to Congress in terms of the incentives that have been put into Hatch-Waxman to encourage early challenges.

For what other purpose was the 180 days implemented but to encourage generic challenges? And so I do not think the Congress—or I do not think the courts have kind of given that deference to the law that has really kind of altered the balance of the way patents work in this particular industry. And it is within Congress's ability, and it is in your right, to alter the patent rights as you see fit.

My last comment is on the 180 days, whether there are suggestions to change it. I think when Congress amended Hatch-Waxman back in 2003 and we had this whole discussion then, I think at the time, talking about whether to go back to the successful defense that the FDA had used or the use it or lose it, I think we can keep the use-it-or-lose approach to the 180 days. I do agree with Mr. Downey in terms of making sure that there is a way to trigger—having a second generic being able to trigger that 180 days so, you know, it does not cause the bottleneck, the 180 does not cause the bottleneck. And I think we have put in our testimony, as I am sure he has in his, ways to amend that 180-day trigger. But I would not amend the entire structure that was settled in 2003.

You know, the one thing I keep kind of looking back at, when Congress looked at that in 2003, the state of the world in terms of these types of settlement agreements was that you had two district courts who had basically said these are per se illegal. You know, these appellate courts in *Tamoxifen* and in the *Schering* case had not yet ruled, and Congress thought the only way to—it is my reading that Congress thought the only way—that we should keep that, that that is a fine balance to have. So the per se rule was actually in effect back in 2003. It is only subsequent events that have changed that through the two court decisions.

So I would leave Hatch-Waxman as it stands with that one amendment to change the trigger to eliminate the bottleneck.

Senator HATCH. Well, if you will recall, the Schumer-McCain bill passed overwhelmingly. It only had one vote against it in the Senate. Guess who that vote was?

Mr. WROBLEWSKI. I do remember, yes.

Senator HATCH. And it never passed. To me it was a great overreach and would have screwed up Hatch-Waxman. This is a very complex bill, but it has worked very, very well. And it took a lot of time to negotiate this and a lot of fights. And one time I threatened to kill all of the people representing PhRMA and the generic industry. I literally did. I had a bad tooth that needed a root canal, and I was in no mood, and they were arguing and yelling around, and I just threatened to kill them all. Frankly, that seemed to bring them together a little bit.

[Laughter.]

Senator HATCH. Mr. Hirsh, you are next.

Mr. HIRSH. Senator Hatch, I guess I should begin by saying I absolutely agree that this is a wonderful piece of legislation and has achieved a great deal, and I am not just saying that because you threaten to kill witnesses.

[Laughter.]

Senator HATCH. Well, I have not threatened you yet.

Mr. HIRSH. Let me address what I think are the points that you are raising and that are being raised in response.

The first issue really relates to a patent being a monopoly, and it goes back to Senator Specter's remarks at the beginning about what did the Eleventh Circuit mean when they had this phrase about, ''exceeding the scope of the patent''.

The difficulty you have in these settlements is the following: Everybody agrees if a patent covers Drug A and you enter into a settlement where you also agree not to compete about Drug B, you are off the reservation. I mean, there is no case that is going to accept that result: that is beyond the scope of the patent. That is not really the issue, and it is not what we are here discussing.

The issue is this: Suppose you have patents where privately, like the example I gave during my oral testimony and in my written testimony about Cephalon, where the companies believe there is a 30-percent chance that the brand company will prevail in this fight—or you can give it another percentage, 40, 50, 60. If the law says you can avoid that fight going to resolution by having the brand company pay the generic to drop the fight, what you are saying is if the cases went to resolution, the brand company would win whatever percentage, 3 out of 10, 4 out of 10—say there are 10 cases, 5 or 6—and they would lose in the remaining number of cases.

Let's take the number 5 for convenience. If you allow the payment from the brand to the generic, you are allowing a situation in which all 10 of those cases result in zero competition and zero benefits for the consumer. If you have those cases go to litigation, you end up with the result that 5 of them expect to come to the result that there is competition and 5 not. If you have a settlement in which they cannot negotiate on the basis of money, but instead have to argue about the length of the time on the patent, you end up with an agreement in which at arm's—length the generic and the brand company have weighed the strength of the patent and come in with a time of entry that reflects the weakness of the patent.

Now, Mr. Downey says, well, we have got these settlements with collateral agreements, and Representative Tauzin gave the example of *Schering-Plough*. *Schering-Plough* is really a good example on the collateral agreements of what I do not understand this legislation to raise as a problem, which is there may well be win-wins between brand and generics on other things. In *Schering-Plough*, there was a cross license. The generics had some drugs under patent, and the brand company—in that case, *Schering-Plough*—paid money and they said, ''We are paying for the cross license.''

Now, there is a factual dispute in the case—and nobody here is going to be able to sort it out—as to whether that was a real payment or not—whether these cross licenses were worth it. But if those cross licenses are worth it, if they are legitimate, that is not a situation where the brand is paying off for the generic. The brand is paying the generic for a license. That is a legitimate deal. And if that is a win-win and that you helps you close the settlement, it helps you close the settlement, and there is nothing that I understand in this bill that necessarily prohibits that. The problem is when the money is not being paid for that. When it is not being paid for some other value, that is what creates the problem.

Now, as for the 180-day provision, that is a glitch in the statute. It is something that should be fixed, but it does not solve this problem for a number of reasons. First of all, even if you have a situation where you can have multiple generics come in to challenge the patent, there is enough money to enter into settlements with all of the generics. That is exactly what happened in *Cephalon*, and there is not—it is in some ways worse to have—five sets of patent litigation settled with reverse payment settlements. It involves more litigation, more payments by the brand company, and no more competition in that scenario than any other scenario. So it does not really address the incentive to do it.

Second, the 180-day provision really does create a special incentive for competition. It is one of the brilliant aspects of the legislation itself. Every other generic manufacturer has less incentive to compete than the one you are settling with if they are the ones holding the 180-day exclusivity provision. So you already enter into a deal that in any other setting—''Pick off your main competitor and pay them not to compete'' are words for an antitrust violation. There is no reason why you should permit that, and so the two are really different problems.

The final point is the alternative of having a court review it. Conceptually, it is a conceivable resolution to the problem. It has some weaknesses. First of all, it does not get you the benefits of a bright-line rule in stopping the lawsuits in the first place and making the process legitimate. And it does not allow, ironically, the market solution of having the arm's-length resolution. Instead what you have is a superimposed solution of what the court thinks a resolution is right. And often per se rules are opposed for the opposite reason. We do not want courts to do that.

But a second basic problem with it is the one that Mr. Wroblewski talked about, which is "what standard should be applied?" It does not solve the entire problem. If you simply say we will have courts look at it, look at it as they did in *Tamoxifen*, look at it as they are going to do in *Cephalon*, who knows what they are going to do with it; look at it as they did in *Schering-Plough*; look at it as they did in *Cardizem*. If the court does not have any guidance to do it, you solve no problem at all by saying let's have the court look at it. The court still needs to be instructed.

Senator HATCH. Well, but one standard by making this a pro se violation—I mean per se, excuse me, violation, that may not work well either.

Mr. HIRSH. I think it does because I think what you are eliminating by the reverse payment is what you want to eliminate. It is a situation in which a payment is the problem. It is not the settlement. Once you eliminate the payment, you have incentivized the brand and generic to reach a competitive settlement, and that is fine. And they can settle by saying, "I have something of value to sell to you, and you are willing to pay for it."

Senator HATCH. So that just creates more litigation.

Mr. HIRSH. No, it does not because, first of all, when—currently under the system, if you have a blockbuster drug, if you have a drug that is selling a billion dollars a year, there is an inherent incentive for a generic company to come up with any argument to file an ANDA-IV. It is true they have to show that it is a bioequivalent. It is not no work at all. But there is a huge incentive to come in there. Why? Because if they can pick any plausible fight at all, they have something that has potential value to it, which is $2 billion of potential sales of a competitor with an awful lot of money to pay off.

Now, any plaintiff's lawyer will tell you if you have got a pot of gold to go after, if you look at securities suits with the market capitalization involved in securities suits, people bring them because there is an enormous amount of money at the end, and far less because there is tremendous merit in every single one of the cases that is being brought. We are incentivizing people to go after that money as opposed to a system that incentivizes people to come in when they really genuinely want to compete and settle the case by agreeing for a time for competition to start. If you take away the payment they will agree they will come in and genuinely compete.

Imagine what would happen to securities litigation if you eliminated a damage remedy. You would not have more litigation. You would have vastly less if you had just injunctive relief.

So the system creates a bad incentive for that type of litigation and less focusing on what the genuine disputes are, less teeing up the right issues for the right dispute with a resolution that harnesses the market.

Senator HATCH. Let me hear from Mr. Tauzin, and I am sorry I have taken so longer here, but these are important questions, and your responses are very important to us.

Mr. TAUZIN. Senator Hatch, Senator Kohl, let me first set some records straight.

One, we are not again generic companies. I am holding up a generic pill made by Teva that I take, that a half-hour before surgery prevented me from having to go through serious surgery this summer on my liver, and I proudly take it every day. It is a good drug. It is a copy of a patented drug that somebody else spent a lot of money to develop, and it is now on the market as a generic, and I am using it. You know, I have got some interest in this as well on a personal level.

Second, we are not just talking about big brand companies and small generic companies. In some cases, we are talking about big generic companies and very small innovators who are members of our association. We have got some companies who just had their first drug approved in our association. And there are lots of small, innovative companies that haven't had their first drug approved, and they have been in business for 10 or 12 years. They are still waiting for that first approval. And so these are contests very often over the patent life of those drugs that involve different size players. It is not just big and little, as you might, you know, think ordinarily.

Third, we are talking about a patent life that the patent holder is entitled to unless his patent is invalid. We are not talking about settlements that extend the patent life beyond what the law gives them. So, you know, you hear comments in here that seem to indicate we are somehow settling cases to keep generic drugs of the market even longer than the patent life that the law allows for the inventor. That is not true. We are simply talking about whether or not the patent life is going to be shortened for the inventor because of a dispute over whether it is a valid patent, done properly, or the new generic company that wants to come in is not infringing. That is a debate. And in those cases, there are issues, obviously, that will yield to settlement rather than to litigation. So that is what we are talking about.

Now, could we help make sure those settlements are in the public interest? Yes, I think there are some ideas that you have discussed today that we would love to talk to you some more about.

I am a little concerned, Senator Hatch, about the 180-day provision. It was one of the beautiful elements of Hatch-Waxman that really encouraged generic companies to come in and test patents.

Senator HATCH. It is a critical element.

Mr. TAUZIN. Yes, and it is part of the balance. That has produced 60-percent generic use in this country, bigger than any country in the world, again. So I would be concerned about messing with it too much.

On the idea of letting the judge who is handling the dispute under whatever standard that makes sense review it, that is worth discussing. That might be an idea that works.

First of all, even Senator Schumer indicated, you know, even though he favors a bright line, he has indicated there are good settlements, and we ought to have some review to see which one is a good one and which one is a bad one. My concern, again, is that if you begin saying what elements of a settlement you cannot ever have, you may make some of these settlements impossible. And, therefore, you may hurt consumers in the end, and you may require small innovators to stay in court longer than they should, at great expense, to protect their patents and, therefore, damage their viability.

You may damage generic companies by forcing them to stay in court longer than they should to get a resolution of the legal issues involved.

So, Senator Hatch, Senator Specter, I respectfully say we would love to sit down and talk some more and visit and see whether there is some other solution. Senator Kohl, I—

Senator HATCH. Well, we would love to hear from all of you.

Mr. TAUZIN. I am just concerned about saying here is an element you cannot have in a settlement just because it looks bad. If it looks bad but it really is good for consumers, maybe the court ought to have the right to say that. If it just looks bad and it is bad, kick it out. It should not be there.

In the end, the judgment ought to be that this helps resolve legal disputes that create uncertainty create legal fights that last too long, cost the companies, cost consumers unnecessarily and in favor of settlements that end these disputes, and let Hatch-Waxman work the way it was intended to by allowing generic companies to enter into the field when they should have a right to be there.

Senator HATCH. Mr. Chairman, I love both sides of the industry and consumers, and, frankly, these matters are not simple matters. This is complex. Hatch-Waxman is complex. There are not too many people that understand it at all in the Congress of the United States. I have to say there are some very good staffers who do in many respects.

But there has been a lot to think about here today, but I have got to tell you these two industries have done so much for America, no question about it. And I get tired of people picking on one or the other, to be honest with you. Both have served this country well.

But there are wrongs, and when there are, current laws many times take care of them. But there needs to be some tinkering here. Even you admit, Mr. Tauzin, that there are bad deals sometimes, and I think you would agree with that, Mr. Downey, as well.

Mr. DOWNEY. We do.

Senator HATCH. And if the law is not taking care of those bad deals, then we have to come up with a way of doing it.

In the case of you, Mr. Wroblewski, and you, Mr. Hirsh, we would like your ideas on this. Personally, I am having some troubles with having a one-size-fits-all answer to this. I have got an open mind on it, and you have certainly—not that I mean that much, but the fact of the matter is that I would like to see if there is some way that we can bring everybody together still in the best interests of the two manufacturers and the consumers as well.

Mr. TAUZIN. Senator, would you indulge me just 1 second longer? I just want to give you an insight that came to me in the last several years since I have been in this job. I have had a chance to go visit a lot of the young scientists working on these new medicines. There is a guy in California, a young scientist working on a medicine for hepatitis B and C, and there are 500 million people on this planet who are going to die from those diseases, about 10 years before they effect on you, kill you. This guy is working on a solution. One guy.

All I am asking you to consider is the long-term effects of what you do in terms of that process, because there are patients all over the world waiting for that scientists and others to invent the drug that eventually the generic companies will copy and bring in at a cheaper cost later on, but who are spending years and years of their life and who dream of nothing else but finding the answer to hepatitis B or C or whatever disease plagues us.

There is a balance here. You talked about it. All we ask is that we make sure this model does not break down, because if it breaks down, for the sake of patients who are currently getting the benefit of a medicine, if we give up what is happening in terms of the incredible research to find the new medicines that are going to take care of those diseases that wreck us and ruin us, that you got to be a little careful that you do not damage that model to the point where it does not work anymore. We are on that brink right.

Senator HATCH. Well, Mr. Chairman, I am sorry I have taken so long, but I do not want either of these industries hurt. There are some people here who think PhRMA is all big businesses. I think you have made a pretty good case that it is a wide variety of businesses, including big businesses. There are some very big generics right now. Yours is one of them, Barr, Teva, a number of others.

In the end, if we hurt these companies by bad legislation, we are going to hurt the consumer in the end. On the other hand, if we allow really what is improper activities to continue—and I have to say I have been pretty forthright about some of what I consider to be improper activities—then we hurt the consumer even more.

So we have to find some way of resolving these problems so that the system works, but we certainly do not want to kill our industry. I love the Washington Post coming out against the House bill over there, which seems to be a political retribution bill more than a bill to protect consumers. And the Post recognized, as I have noticed they do, they recognize that we do not want to kill these industries. We are the leaders in the world today, and our hope for the future of controlling health care costs is going to be just how successful you folks are and what we can do with stem cell research and bio as we go down through the years. And if we are successful in those, especially bio and stem cell research, if we are successful in individual therapies based upon genetics for individual people, I got to tell you, we might be able to avoid an awful lot of Medicaid and Medicare costs that are going to swamp the Federal budget in the future unless we can find some ways around it.

So I want to commend you for the work that you do, and I am sorry I have taken so long, but—actually, you have taken most of the time. I have just been very reasonable.

[Laughter.]

Senator HATCH. But this has been an extremely interesting hearing to me, and I just want to compliment all of you, and compliment you, Mr. Chairman. I am going to really enjoy working with you, as I always have, and this is a very important hearing, and I hope we will hold some others as well on other matters.

Senator KOHL. Thank you for your contribution, Senator Hatch.

Senator Grassley?

STATEMENT OF CHARLES E. GRASSLEY, A U.S. SENATOR FROM THE STATE OF IOWA

Senator GRASSLEY. Mr. Chairman, I am not going to ask any questions. First of all, I did not think I was going to be able to be here at all. I am very interested in this subject and am a cosponsor of the bill, but I was working with Senator Baucus to get a small business tax provision out of the Finance Committee, which we just got done, so it would be ready for the minimum wage bill. But now that this Committee was still meeting, I wanted to stop by and let everybody know that I am going to continue working with the Chairman of the Committee and other members of this Committee on this legislation. I think it is needed. I would not preclude the possibility of compromise and listening to every point of view as just expressed by Senator Hatch. But I think there is a lot in this area that needs to be done, and I think the most important thing is to make sure that the marketplace works and is not frustrated from the standpoint of when patents have expired, we ought to expect generics to get to market as soon as possible.

So in the process of doing that, I wanted to stop by and express my support and regret why I could not be here for the entire hearing. I will have a chance to be briefed on everything that was said. And I assume that it is Chairman Leahy's intent to move ahead with this legislation. I, at least, hope so.

So I thank Senator Leahy and you for your work and for putting my statement in the record. Thank you.

[The prepared statement of Senator Grassley appears as a submission for the record.]

Senator KOHL. Thank you very much, Senator Grassley.

Gentlemen, we appreciate your being here, as well as Commissioner Leibowitz. This has been a very good hearing on a very complicated and a very important topic. You have shed a lot of light with your discussion this morning. We appreciate the time you have given us and the wisdom that you have brought to the issue. Thank you so much.

The hearing is adjourned.

[Whereupon, at 12:10 p.m., the Committee was adjourned.]

[Questions and answers and submissions for the record follow.]

In: Generic Drugs: Needs and Issues
Editor: Ryan S. Blanton

ISBN: 978-1-60692-843-1
© 2009 Nova Science Publishers, Inc.

Chapter 3

SAFE AND AFFORDABLE BIOTECH DRUGS: THE NEED FOR A GENERIC PATHWAY[*]

The committee met, pursuant to notice, at 10 a.m., in room 2154, Rayburn House Office Building, Hon. Henry A. Waxman (chairman of the committee) presiding.

Present: Representatives Waxman, Kucinich, Davis of Illinois, Yarmuth, Norton, Van Hollen, Hodes, Welch, Davis of Virginia, Burton, Issa, Bilbray, and Sali.

Staff present: Phil Barnett, staff director and chief counsel; Kristin Amerling, general counsel; Karen Nelson, health policy director; Karen Lightfoot, communications director and senior policy advisor; Andy Schneider, chief health counsel; Sarah Despres, senior health counsel; Ann Witt, health counsel; Robin Appleberry and Rachel Sher, counsels; Earley Green, chief clerk; Teresa Coufal, deputy clerk; Caren Auchman, press assistant; Zhongrui ''JR'' Deng, chief information officer; Leneal Scott, information systems manager; Robin Pam, staff assistant; David Marin, minority staff director; Larry Halloran, minority deputy staff director; Jennifer Safavian, minority chief counsel for oversight and investigations; Susie Schulte, minority senior professional staff member; Kristina Husar, minority professional staff member; Patrick Lyden, minority parliamentarian and member services coordinator; Brian McNicoll, minority communications director; and Benjamin Chance, minority clerk.

---

[*] This is an edited, reformatted and augmented version of a Hearing before the Committee on Oversight and Government Reform, House of Representatives, One Hundred Tenth Congress, First Session, on March 26, 2007, Serial No. 110-43.

Chairman WAXMAN. The meeting of the committee will please come to order.

More than 20 years ago the Congress enacted the Hatch-Waxman Act. That law has taught us three things: genetic drugs are good for patients, both medically and financially; with a little help, the market works, generic competition lowers drug prices; and generic competition does not bankrupt the brand name drug industry or slow innovation.

Maybe some big drug makers still dispute these lessons, but no one else does. But there is still no generic competition for one of the fastest-growing and most expensive categories of drugs, biologicals, those drugs produced from living cell cultures rather than from chemical synthesis.

Some of these drugs are near miracles for people with cancer, metabolic diseases, and immune disorders. They can stop disability and, in some cases, save lives. People need them. But some of these drugs cost each patient tens of thousands of dollars a year. Some can cost hundreds of thousands per year. Many people cannot get access to these near miracles, and even when people can get them the prices drive up the cost of Medicare, Medicaid, and health insurance overall.

Why isn't the market helping? It is not because of the patent system that biologicals are protected from the competition that might lower prices. Biologicals, like other drugs, do enjoy patent protection. This allows manufacturers to enjoy a monopoly period during which they can get a significant return on their investments. But patents, or many of them, have already expired, and other patents are just about to expire.

And it is not the science of these drugs that protects them from competition. The technology is already here to make a safe and effective copy of some biotech drugs. Moreover, the technology is getting better every year, and we can make progress even faster if we allow companies to use it to make generics.

Instead, the monopoly on each of these drugs is perpetuated by the lack of a clear pathway for FDA to approve competing versions.

The Hatch-Waxman Act does not reach most of them. This costs all of us—taxpayers, insurance premium payers, and patients—billions of dollars. It also means that some very sick people simply cannot get the drugs they need.

I know that the science of these drugs is not simple. I take the questions of research, safety, and efficacy very seriously. The only way we can succeed in establishing robust competition for biotech drugs is with drugs the doctors and patients know they can count on, so we need to be sure that the FDA has the discretion to require the studies that are needed to establish that a copy of a biotech drug is equivalent to the brand name drug in safety and effectiveness. That is one of the things we hope to learn more about today.

But the big brand name companies have gone beyond legitimate concern and have thrown up a defensive smoke screen around biologicals. They say there will be problems of safety, decreased innovation, and limited savings. When discussing creating generic competition, they say things like, ''Such action may also save consumers a few dollars here and there, although that is by no means assured, but whatever short-term savings may be achieved will come at an enormous long-term cost to the public. Focusing solely upon short-term, lower prices, a cheap drugs policy will inevitably reduce research and hinder our public health efforts.''

Well, these arguments have a familiar ring to them. That is because the words I just read were the formal testimony that the Pharmaceutical Manufacturers Association gave to the House in 1983 when they were opposing Hatch-Waxman, and now manufacturers are using these same arguments again. But they were wrong then. Hatch-Waxman has saved patients billions of dollars and dramatically improved their access to drugs, and Hatch-Waxman did not reduce research or hinder public health.

And they are wrong now. A new path for FDA to approve generic biologicals will save patients billions in the future and will improve access to treatments and cures, and a new path will improve competition, while preserving the market's strong incentive for research.

For the sake of patients, their families, public and private health insurance, and taxpayers, we must find a way to introduce competition to this market. When a patent expires, we owe it to consumers to find a way through competition to lower prices and still deliver a safe and effective product. When a patient expires, they no longer need the product, so the price will make no difference.

I look forward to the testimony of the witnesses today and learning more about the scope of the problem, the science, and the potential solutions.

[The prepared statement of Chairman Henry A. Waxman follows:]

Chairman WAXMAN. Mr. Davis.

Mr. DAVIS OF VIRGINIA. Thank you, Mr. Chairman, for holding today's hearing to consider the implications of creating a regulatory pathway for approval of follow-on biologics. It is a very important subject, and certainly your leadership is appreciated and worthy of this committee's consideration.

Mr. Chairman, you have long been a leader in improving access to pharmaceutical drugs. Indeed, there is near universal agreement that the Hatch-Waxman Act has been extremely effective in allowing generic drugs to come to market and compete with brand name drugs. This competition has benefited countless citizens, as well as the Federal Government, by using natural market economics to bring down the price of prescription medicine. You are to be commended for your leadership in improving access to these life-saving medications.

It is my understanding you have recently introduced legislation that would, in fact, create a regulatory pathway for the FDA to approve follow-on biologics. We have been reviewing the legislation with interest, and we expect it will inform today's discussion.

I look forward to exploring your proposal further. For now, let me just offer a few preliminary thoughts on this very complex subject.

The first principle guiding this effort should be to foster innovation and the discovery of new cures. After all, there is no new therapeutic, by definition there can be no follow-on. Accordingly, we need to protect the intellectual property of innovative firms. Given the high cost of research, development, manufacturing, and regulatory approvals, IP protections are clearly a critical factor for biotech startups when they are securing venture capital and pursuing partnerships with larger firms.

Today we will hear from economist Henry Grabowski, who will explain that increased patent uncertainty and IP litigation would have a significant negative effect on capital market decisions for emerging private and public biotech firms. He will explain that if the Federal Government either weakens patent protections or increases the chance of litigation there will likely be a corresponding decrease in investment, and therefore less research and development of biologics. It would be tragic if legislation intended to increase access to medicine would have the unintended result of stifling innovation, preventing the discovery of cures of presently terminal diseases.

I hope you would agree with me, Mr. Chairman, about the importance of fostering a vibrant and innovative culture where we encourage our brightest minds and daring entrepreneurs to do the research, provide the investment so that we may some day discover the cure for cancer or Lou Gehrig's disease.

Reflecting on the Hatch-Waxman Act, you got it right when you recognized the importance of balancing the twin goals of bringing generic drugs to market while at the same time leaving intact the financial incentive for research and development.

One of the keys to this successful balance in that legislation was the guarantee of 5 years of market exclusivity for innovative companies. Incidentally, European Union regulators currently provide 10 years of market exclusivity for European drugs for innovative drugs. Some amount of market exclusivity for the innovator is necessary under any regulatory pathway for follow-on biologics.

The second imperative is to provide a mechanism so the FDA is able to guarantee the safety and efficacy of follow-on biologics. To do so we have to recognize the fundamental differences between biologics and chemical-based pharmaceuticals. What has proven to be successful in the case of traditional drugs is not necessary transferrable to the science of biologics. For instance, it is currently possible to know the complete character of a small molecule drug. This knowledge enables the FDA to approve generic drugs with the same characteristics as the innovator drug without requiring generic companies to test and prove the drug's efficacy and safety again. However, current science has not advanced sufficiently to give us the same confidence that a follow-on biologic is identical to a previously approved biologic based on molecular structure, alone.

Unlike traditional drugs, which are chemically based, biologics are made from living organisms. Even minor variations in manufacturing processes can have a significant impact on the final character and consistency of the biologic and its effect on the human body.

This diagram on the board comparing a biologic used to treat anemia and a traditional drug that treats peptic ulcers disease demonstrates the difference between traditional chemical drugs and biological therapies. As you can see, the biologic is significantly more complex than a traditional drug, having a molecular weight of 30,000 versus 351. This is a critical distinction between traditional generic drugs and follow-on biologics. Any regulatory pathway must take full account of this distinction, which for now seems to point to the inescapable conclusion that clinical trials on some level will be essential to ensure the safety and efficacy of followon biological products.

Again I want to thank you, Mr. Chairman, for spurring a discussion on this important subject. I look forward to hearing from our distinguished panel of witnesses.

[The prepared statement of Hon. Tom Davis follows:]

Chairman WAXMAN. Thank you very much, Mr. Davis.

Without objection, all Members will be permitted to enter an opening statement in the record. Do any Members wish, however, to make any comments before we hear from our 15 witnesses? Mr. Issa.

Mr. ISSA. Thank you, Mr. Chairman. I will be brief. I will put my formal statement in the record, particularly because it sounds an awful lot like Mr. Davis'. The view is somewhat the same, and that is that it is very clear that we know a great deal about chemical compounds and we can say a chemical is a chemical, but, for example, Mr. Chairman, would you want to have these two oranges substituted as though there were no difference? Would you accept that a Florida orange is the same as a California orange if you have to peel it, Mr. Chairman? And, for Mr. Sali who is not here today, do you really think that any

Russett potato is an Idaho potato and should be interchanged and have no value, no second testing of whether or not it makes a good french fry?

Now, clearly we know how to make grain alcohol, and if I am buying grain alcohol, Mr. Chairman, it is very clear that I know that it is alcohol plus about 3 percent water that just gets in if you get the air to it. But, Mr. Chairman, do you really think that a $90 bottle of California wine that says Merlot is equal to this fine boxed Merlot? And would you want to go to the dinner table or the hospital and have them interchanged without your prior approval, or perhaps a little taste?

This is biologics. These are made by process. Mr. Chairman, they may both be a Merlot, but as a Californian, I am sure that you would not want them interchanged without your prior approval.

With that, I yield back.

[The prepared statement of Hon. Darrell E. Issa follows:]

Chairman WAXMAN. Mr. Davis.

Mr. DAVIS OF ILLINOIS. Yes, Mr. Chairman, I would like to make a brief statement.

Chairman WAXMAN. Before I recognize you for that purpose, I would like to inquire if you have any props. [Laughter.]

The gentleman is recognized.

Mr. DAVIS OF ILLINOIS. Thank you very much, Mr. Chairman. I shall, indeed, be brief. But first of all let me thank you for calling this hearing.

In 1984 the landmark Hatch-Waxman Act provided a cost-effective alternative to branded drugs with the creation of a traditional generic pharmaceutical industry. Today's hearing marks yet another landmark as we are being called upon to address escalating biopharmaceutical costs.

This issue is near and dear to me, one, as a former health administrator, but also because my congressional district has more hospitals and more hospital beds than any other congressional district in the country. Illinois has about 200 hospitals, most of them nonprofit. State hospitals are losing money, and another third are barely breaking even, notwithstanding cuts in Medicare and Medicaid.

According to Crane's Chicago Business, on February 13, 2006, while the State of Illinois has implemented prescription drug assistance programs like the Senior Care Pharmaceutical Program, State Pharmaceutical Assistance Plan, All Kids Program that provides health insurance coverage and prescription drugs to children across all socio-economic groups, they help to buffer costs.

However, the sad reality is that cuts in Federal spending tend to shift costs to insured patients and their employers. By definition, health care is eating up a piece of our income, which is especially bad news for the 26 percent of Chicagoans, including 164,203 with full-time jobs and 43,876 with at least a college education who lack health insurance. These data are particularly disturbing when you take into consideration the median household income for Chicago is $38,625 a year.

With this in mind, I welcome today's distinguished panelists and look forward to their insight and recommendations on how we can buildupon the foundation of generic competition for our consumers laid some 23 years ago under the Hatch-Waxman Act toward the attainment of a pathway to safe and affordable biotech drugs.

I guess if I was to have any kind of prop, I'd just take this water, which is pretty pure, and be delighted to have it.

Again, thank you, Mr. Chairman, for having this hearing.

Chairman WAXMAN. Thank you very much, Mr. Davis.

Does any other Member wish to be recognized for an opening statement? Mr. Yarmuth.

Mr. YARMUTH. Mr. Chairman, two things real briefly. First of all, I hope that Mr. Issa would accept an amendment to his list in saying that no self-respecting Kentuckian would accept Tennessee sour mash whiskey for a Kentucky bourbon.

Mr. ISSA. Now that is bipartisan if I ever saw it.

Mr. YARMUTH. Thank you.

Also, I would like to say that I think the chairman and Mr. Davis have very accurately expressed and illuminated the conflicting issues that we have to deal with on this topic.

I would also mention the fact that we have to recognize that much of the research that leads to the development of these drugs and these medications, both pharmaceutical and also these biologics, are funded by taxpayer dollars initially, so that we have an overriding mandate to do what is best for the taxpayer, who is paying for most of this research at the very foundational levels.

Thank you, Mr. Chairman.

Chairman WAXMAN. Thank you very much.

We will now hear from our witnesses today. Our first witness I am pleased to welcome is Dr. Janet Woodcock. She is the Deputy Commissioner for Operations and Chief Medical Officer of the Food and Drug Administration.

Since you are standing, I will have you continue to stand because it is the practice of this committee to put all witnesses under oath. [Witness sworn.]

Chairman WAXMAN. The record will indicate that you answered in the affirmative.

We are delighted to have you here. We will put your full statement in the record. If it is possible, we would like to ask you to keep to around 5 minutes.

STATEMENT OF JANET WOODCOCK, M.D., DEPUTY COMMISSIONER FOR OPERATIONS AND CHIEF MEDICAL OFFICER, FOOD AND DRUG ADMINISTRATION

Dr. WOODCOCK. Thank you. Mr. Chairman and members of the committee, I am Janet Woodcock, Deputy Commissioner and Chief Medical Officer of the Food and Drug Administration. I thank you for the opportunity to testify about the scientific and regulatory framework surrounding follow-on biologics.

In considering the complex scientific issues at hand, I have relied not only on my experience leading the Center for Drug Evaluation and Research for over a decade, but also on my 8 years of experience working in the Center for Biologics Evaluation and Research [CBER]. While in CBER I served as Acting Deputy Center Director and as Director of the Office of Therapeutics, in which capacity I oversaw the approval of biotechnology products to treat serious illnesses such as cancer, multiple sclerosis, and cystic fibrosis.

The success of FDA's generic drugs program has spurred interest in considering abbreviated application pathways for more-complex molecules. Currently there are over 9,000 approved therapeutically equivalent generic drugs on the market. They constitute about 60 percent of prescriptions written in the United States. FDA's Office of Generic Drugs currently approves generics at the rate of more than one per calendar day.

The success of the program has stimulated competition. For the last decade, the rate of submission to the Office of Generic Drugs has rapidly increased. Submissions doubled between 2002 and 2006, to a current rate of about 793 applications per year.

The office has implemented numerous process improvements, have improved increased efficiency of the review process, and recently, as part of FDA's initiative on pharmaceutical quality for the 21st century, OGD instituted the question-based review. Eventually it is hoped this change will decrease submission of manufacturing supplements by about 80 percent, and thus free up more time of the reviewers to deal with this increased submission rate.

While the generics program has been very successful for small molecules, scientific challenges remain. We do not have good bioequivalents methods for inhaled or many topical medications, and must require clinical trials to demonstrate equivalence. This has inhibited consumer access to generic versions of these types of products.

In addition, a number of drugs are made from complex molecules. In these cases, it can be difficult to tell whether a proposed generic version is structurally identical to the innovator product.

Recently, as part of its critical path initiative, FDA has been evaluating the science needed to address these issues for generic drugs and is planning to lay out the scientific research that is needed to improve the process, as we did a number of years ago for innovator medical products.

The topic for discussion today is variously referred to as followon proteins, follow-on biologics, generic biologics, as well as other labels. Many of these terms are very imprecise and confusing, and I hope we can discuss terminology.

Largely, these terms are intended to refer to biotechnology produced protein products. In the United States, such products are regulated either as drugs under the Food, Drug, and Cosmetic Act, or as biologic products under the Public Health Service Act. Whether regulated as drugs or biologic products, proteins fit into the category of complex molecules that can be difficult to fully characterize.

Copies of protection products that are regulated as drugs may be considered for the abbreviated applications pathways that exist under section 505. The very simplest peptide products may be able to demonstrate that they contain the same active ingredient as the innovator product, and thus may be considered under 505(j), what is commonly regarded as the generic drug pathway.

In contrast, copies of approved protein products that are drugs would currently be considered for abbreviated applications under 505(b)(2), and the reason for this is that scientific techniques are not available to demonstrate sameness of these types of molecules.

The degree to which any abbreviated pathway could be used for any given protein depends on many factors, including its physical complexity, the availability of functional assays to characterize it, and its clinical use.

An abbreviated pathway does not exist for copies of protein products approved under the PHS Act. FDA has approved several follow-on proteins under 505(b)(2), including a recombinant hyaluronidase and recombinant version of human growth hormone.

We are currently preparing a guidance document on the general scientific framework for preparation of abbreviated applications for follow-on proteins under 505(b)(2). We expect to follow this with guidance on technical issues such as immunogenicity, dealing with immunogenicity of proteins and physical characterization methods.

I will be pleased to answer your questions regarding these complex issues.

[The prepared statement of Dr. Woodcock follows:]

Chairman WAXMAN. Thank you very much, Dr. Woodcock.

As you mention in your testimony, for over 10 years FDA has allowed brand name manufacturers of biotech drugs to make certain changes in the process by which they manufacture their products, but without repeating all the original clinical trials, under something called comparability protocols. I am interested in understanding the scientific rationale for allowing brand name manufacturers to make process changes without new clinical trials. I am also interested in its applicability to follow-on and biogeneric products.

What was the scientific basis for FDA's conclusion that clinical outcome trials are not necessary to assess the effects of certain biological product changes?

Dr. WOODCOCK. Manufacturing changes and process changes are undertaken for all pharmaceutical products, whether drugs or biologics. In each case we have to determine whether or not the change could result in any clinically significant change in the product, whether it is a small molecule or whether it is a large, complex molecule of some kind. FDA has a long history of quality regulation, putting into place procedures, both physical characterization of the new product and comparing it to the old product, functional characterization of a new product compared to the original product, and sometimes clinical characterization of a new product. It depends on, as I said in my oral testimony, how much science we have available to assess these changes.

If we can be sure, based on a structural characterization, which we often can for a drug, then that would be sufficient for a small molecule drug. If that structural characterization isn't enough to assure that the new version is similar to the old version, then other types of tests might be necessary. And in some cases we might even require clinical tests.

For example, with small molecule drugs, when the formulation is changed we may require new bioequivalent studies.

Chairman WAXMAN. So that is completely within your discretion based on whether you think it is appropriate to have further evaluations, further studies?

Dr. WOODCOCK. Yes. There are multiple scientific issues that come into play in any given manufacturing change.

Chairman WAXMAN. I know most of these comparability decisions involving biotech drugs or any other drugs are confidential, but with the biotech drug Avonex the information is public. I assume you are familiar with that case?

Dr. WOODCOCK. Yes.

Chairman WAXMAN. What kinds of process changes did FDA permit in that case without repeating the original safety and effectiveness trials?

Dr. WOODCOCK. In that case the original cell line that had been used to manufacture the product that was used in the clinical trials was no longer available, so the manufacturer had to go back and redo all of that and duplicate the manufacturing process that had been used for the original product. That is well described publicly. They made some original attempts. Those weren't successful.

They made some subsequent attempts and then an extensive number of comparisons were made between the original product and the second version of the product, both the kinds I just described, both physical/chemical comparisons, functional comparisons, and so forth, so that at the end of the day it was decided that the products were similar enough that FDA could extrapolate from the clinical data that was derived for the first product to the new product.

Chairman WAXMAN. Were the changes between the two products significant?

Dr. WOODCOCK. The products were very similar, ended up being very similar.

Chairman WAXMAN. I meant the process changes. Were they significant?

Dr. WOODCOCK. The manufacturer attempted to duplicate the similar process that was originally done with the first product, but it was in a different site, in a different scale, and so forth, so there were differences. It was not the identical cell line. It wasn't the identical product that had been made, and so forth.

Chairman WAXMAN. Are these changes similar to the kinds of changes that might be required to manufacture a follow-on product?

Dr. WOODCOCK. The difference between that example and the instance where a new manufacturer would attempt to manufacture a follow-on product would be that in the Avonex case. The manufacturer had access to all the information about the process of manufacturing the first product. That is very important information, because it has information on all the intermediate steps and what happens during the manufacturing and purification process, and so on.

Chairman WAXMAN. Thank you.

Mr. Davis.

Mr. DAVIS OF VIRGINIA. We will start with Mr. Issa.

Chairman WAXMAN. Mr. Issa.

Mr. ISSA. Thank you. Thank you, Mr. Chairman, and thank you, Ranking Member Davis.

Avonex appears to be an example sort of—I will use a different wine than the one here, but you are talking if the Rothschilds trying to duplicate after they have had to clear their grapes away and put a new crop in. You have the same maker with the same wine masters—in this case scientists—trying to duplicate what they had already made. Is that roughly correct? You may not be a California wine drinker, so I know it can be challenging.

Dr. WOODCOCK. I love California wine.

Mr. ISSA. You won't love the one here in this box. Trust me.

Dr. WOODCOCK. Yes. As an analogy, that is quite reasonable.

Mr. Issa. OK. So the next step that the chairman's legislation or the legislation we are hearing here today would attempt to do is to say that, even though you had to sort of teach or go through a process, a re-learning process, even with the original designer, you are going to try and transfer this to a different winery, and they are going to try to set up, but they are not going to have the right to every trade secret, if you will. Not every nuance of the process is, in fact, in the public domain. Is that correct?

Dr. Woodcock. That is correct. We face that now with our generic drug program.

Mr. Issa. OK. And you mentioned earlier that you have had chemical equivalents that didn't work out so well when they went generic, so to speak, even among name manufacturers. When an insurance company does a formulary and says this is equal to this, that is not always right, is it? There are side effects that are unanticipated often?

Dr. Woodcock. The generic drugs that we approve are fully interchangeable with the innovator drugs. They are therapeutically equivalent.

Mr. Issa. You have never had a side effect?

Dr. Woodcock. We have numerous reports of side effects; however, we investigate those and we have extraordinarily rarely found any instance where there would be therapeutic inequivalence between a generic drug and an innovator drug.

Mr. Issa. Now, when we get to biological and follow-on immune problems that occur, that is a different problem that you are not presently seeing as much in small cells but you do see it in biologics, don't you?

Dr. Woodcock. Yes. Proteins are what is called immunogenic. They produce often an immune response in people when they are administered.

Mr. Issa. So if there are two otherwise the same biologies, the original and the follow-on, one could very much have a different immune response that would lead somebody who had successfully fought a disease to somehow develop a resistance; is that correct?

Dr. Woodcock. The immune response to a protein can cause many things. It can cause what you just said, which is neutralizing the effect, the beneficial effect of the protein.

Mr. Issa. And then you could find yourself unable to deal with either drug. In other words, you could make that change and find yourself opted out of the cure or the treatment?

Dr. Woodcock. That is true, and there are difficulties, for example, with insulin sometimes.

Mr. Issa. So, given that you have this history, wouldn't, in the case of follow-on biologics, at least until this problem can be quantified, wouldn't you have a bias, an almost exclusive bias toward clinical trials, even if we gave you the jurisdiction and the right to shortcut those, limit those, eliminate them? From a standpoint of unsettled science, wouldn't it be proper to have clinical trials to ensure that is not happening when, in fact, it can take someone who is surviving and put them in a position where they can no longer survive?

Dr. Woodcock. Currently—and, of course, I can only address the proteins that we are looking at under the 505, under the FD&C Act.

Mr. Issa. Right, and you admit those are, by definition, less likely to be unknowns than the ones we are going toward; is that right?

Dr. Woodcock. No. That is where the terminology I think is very confusing. We have approved proteins under the Food, Drug and Cosmetic Act provisions under 505(b)(2), and in those cases, for those recombinant proteins we have looked at the immunogenicity in people.

Mr. Issa. OK, but you have looked at them?

Dr. Woodcock. Yes.

Mr. Issa. So, again, my one final exit question here in this short time: clinical trials are the only way to know whether substantially similar, substantially identical follow-on biologics are, in fact, going to have differences in the immune response, or whatever term is appropriate; is that right?

Dr. Woodcock. Yes. We have a very limited understanding of the basis of an immune response, and we are not able to fully predict immunogenicity in humans right now from non-clinical data.

Mr. Issa. And this could be dangerous?

Dr. Woodcock. The immunogenicity must be evaluated.

Mr. Issa. Thank you, Mr. Chairman.

Chairman Waxman. Thank you, Mr. Issa.

Mr. Yarmuth.

Mr. Yarmuth. Thank you, Mr. Chairman.

Dr. Woodcock, some in the brand name industry argue that any process for approving copies of biologics should follow the European Union model. The EU's governing directive, which is comparable to a statute, is extremely flexible and gives regulators great discretion to set procedures and standards and so forth.

The drug regulatory body there, the EMEA, has also established very particular procedures and approval standards to implement those directives. You are nodding, so you are obviously familiar with that process or that model?

Dr. Woodcock. Yes.

Mr. YARMUTH. And the biotech industry seems to like that public process that is used there for establishing and setting guidelines that contain the data requirements for biosimilars because the data gathering process allows those companies to help dictate what data their competitors must produce, and, of course, that would take a lengthy period of time.

Is the FDA required to undertake a public process for establishing data requirements?

Dr. WOODCOCK. No. We are not required to.

Mr. YARMUTH. Do you think it is scientifically necessary for FDA to engage in a public guideline process to establish the data requirements for a follow-on protein product?

Dr. WOODCOCK. What FDA does currently is engage with the manufacturer in discussions—of course, those are not public—to provide advice on any manufacturer interested in pursuing a follow-on under the 505(b)(2) process. But we often write scientific guidance for manufacturers because it provides better predictability and it provides, as you said, transparency.

We are in the process of writing overall guidance on the process of scientific approach to follow-on proteins under 505(b)(2).

Mr. YARMUTH. Do you think that the process the European Union uses, if we adopted that system here, would have the effect of freezing science at all? Is that a risk in doing that?

Dr. WOODCOCK. I am really not able to comment on that.

Mr. YARMUTH. Thank you, Mr. Chairman. I yield back.

Chairman WAXMAN. The gentleman has a couple minutes, would you yield your time to me?

Mr. YARMUTH. I would be happy to yield my time to the distinguished chairman.

Chairman WAXMAN. Thank you.

I just wanted to point out that the questioning by my colleague, Mr. Issa, about how you might need to have clinical trials to understand possible concerns, that is legitimate. FDA does now at the present time allow some changes in the process without requiring clinical trials, but I do want to point out that the legislation that I have introduced would allow FDA to decide, when they think clinical trials are appropriate, to require clinical trials.

I do want to ask you this. In the use of comparability protocols limited to simple proteins, can the manufactures of more complex proteins make changes in their products without repeating the original clinical trials?

Dr. WOODCOCK. Yes, they can, if the science is there. It is very desirable for manufacturers of pharmaceuticals of any kind to make continuous improvements in their manufacturing process to maintain the quality of the pharmaceuticals as soon as possible and the efficiency of the process as good as scientifically possible. So FDA has adopted procedures, as I said, that allow manufacturers to make changes to their manufacturing process or perhaps open up new plants, say, if there is a demand for the product, and the amount of data that has to be generated really depends on the complexity of the product, how well we can physically characterize the product, and how confident we are that physical characterization will extrapolate to the same performance. But we may require many additional steps, up to and including clinical studies now, particularly of immunogenicity.

Chairman WAXMAN. Well, do you and other FDA scientists feel confident that comparability assessments provide adequate protection to patients from unsafe or ineffective biotech drugs?

Dr. WOODCOCK. The comparability assessment puts the burden on the manufacturer. The manufacturer must show to FDA's satisfaction that the change has not introduced anything that would be detrimental to the clinical performance of the drug. So how much evidence is needed after a manufacturing change depends on how well the manufacturer can demonstrate that product is going to perform the exact same way as the original product did in the clinical testing.

Chairman WAXMAN. And as science evolves, you will know better whether the comparability requires clinical tests or not; is that correct?

Dr. WOODCOCK. The ability to physically characterize protein molecules and other complex substances has evolved and is continuing to evolve, and so over time we are going to be able to do a better and better job of controlling the quality of these products and allowing for continuous improvement.

Chairman WAXMAN. Thank you very much.

Mr. Davis.

Mr. DAVIS OF VIRGINIA. I finally have my comparison up there. We talked before about how complex these are. This diagram up there, as you see, compares a biologic used to treat anemia and a traditional drug that treats peptic ulcers. It demonstrates the difference between the traditional chemical drugs and biological therapies.

Dr. WOODCOCK. Yes.

Mr. DAVIS OF VIRGINIA. As you can note on this, the biologic is significantly more complex than a traditional drug.

Dr. Woodcock, you highlight in your testimony the importance of ensuring that facilitating the development of follow-on products through abbreviated pathways doesn't discourage innovation and the development of new biological products, and you refer to Hatch-Waxman as a balanced approach. Do you think an extended period of data exclusivity as well as certain patent protections like Hatch-Waxman would help encourage innovation and development with biological products?

Dr. WOODCOCK. Sir, I am a doctor and a scientist, and that is really outside of my area of expertise.

Mr. DAVIS OF VIRGINIA. OK, so you don't want to make the economic or policy determinations on that? Dr. WOODCOCK. No. Mr. DAVIS OF VIRGINIA. OK. You also state in your testimony that demonstrating the similarity of a follow-on protein product to a reference product is more complex and would require new data. Does this mean FDA would require clinical safety data for followon biologics?

Dr. WOODCOCK. There is a very large range of complexity. All right? The erythropoietin molecule that you have here is a pretty complex example. There are very, very small biologic drugs of different kinds. So the amount of assurance and the amount of data that would be needed is really based on how complex something is and how well it can be characterized in different ways.

Mr. DAVIS OF VIRGINIA. But a slight alteration could have, you know, significant clinical manifestations, wouldn't it?

Dr. WOODCOCK. FDA would not approve a follow-on product or a generic drug that we were not confident would have the same performance as the innovator drug.

Mr. DAVIS OF VIRGINIA. What level of clinical safety data would be necessary for approval, ball park?

Dr. WOODCOCK. Well, to talk about this we have to get into terminology a little bit. Please bear with me.

The abbreviated application process for 505(b)(2), for example, may rely on some fact of the approval of a prior product. All right?

Mr. DAVIS OF VIRGINIA. Yes.

Dr. WOODCOCK. But we may approve a product using an abbreviated application where some of the data, maybe some of the clinical trials or animal studies do not have to be repeated. However, that resulting of proof product is not considered substitutable for the other product. In other words, each of them stand alone and they can't be switched at the pharmacy, or it is not recommended they would be. That is one level.

Another level would be for a manufacturer to seek interchangeability, full interchangeability. So far the proteins that we have approved all stand on their own. They have had abbreviated applications but they are not considered interchangeable with any of the other proteins in that class. For example, human growth hormone or hyaluronidase.

Mr. DAVIS OF VIRGINIA. You testified that the science and technology isn't sufficiently advanced to allow for comparison of complex protein products. How close are we to discovering those technology methods; 5 years; 10 years?

Dr. WOODCOCK. It is going to be a continuum, and right now we are very short peptides, which are as small as the ranidine molecule you are showing there, for example, or in the same ball park. We can do it now, but those are very, very small compared to the erythropoietin molecule, so it is going to be a step-wise progression over a decade or so.

Mr. DAVIS OF VIRGINIA. Are there any non-clinical tests or technology that could fully substitute for studying the safety of biotech products in humans?

Dr. WOODCOCK. As I said, right now we do not have the science around the immune system to adequately predict the human immune response fully to any given product.

Mr. DAVIS OF VIRGINIA. You listed two examples, omnitrope and—I can't pronounce the other one. Hyaluronidase?

Dr. WOODCOCK. That is pretty good.

Mr. DAVIS OF VIRGINIA. Neither was rated by FDA as therapeutically equivalent or substitutes for other biologics on the market. Many believe interchangeability or substitution is where the most cost savings would occur. Of course, the balance here is safety versus efficiency and speed to market.

When do you think the FDA will be able to rate a biologic product as interchangeable? And do you think the FDA needs this authority if the science isn't developed yet?

Dr. WOODCOCK. For the 505(b)(2) drugs, which is what I can comment on, manufacturers would need to do additional clinical studies that would demonstrate interchangeability, and that is a further step. That is a higher bar than simply getting on the market, an abbreviated application. Does that make sense to you?

Chairman WAXMAN. Thank you, Mr. Davis.

Mr. Welch.

Mr. WELCH. Thank you, Mr. Chairman.

Some of the drug companies have said that when a biotech product is derived from a specific cell line, any copy of the product will have to begin with a different cell line. They are arguing, as I understand it, that this change is so significant that all the clinical trials, all the clinical trials must be repeated to ensure that the change has not altered safety and effectiveness. Obviously, we are concerned about safety, but we also want to get the benefit and not have this argument about safety be used to deny us the benefit.

My question to you is: is it true that a change in a cell line will always necessitate repeating the original clinical trials?

Dr. WOODCOCK. No. We do not believe that. Again, any manufacturing change, whether the cell line, the DNA construct, the manufacturing process, the way the drug is purified, any of these could affect safety and effectiveness, and therefore data has to be submitted and a very careful look has to be taken to make sure that it hasn't. The amount of data that we would need or that anyone would need to make that evaluation depends, again, on the complexity of the product.

Mr. WELCH. All right. So the bottom line here is that you believe that you do not need, for safety, to repeat the entire clinical trial?

Dr. WOODCOCK. In some instances the manufacturer may not be able to show enough similarity and they may have to repeat much of the clinical program. In other instances they may be able to show an extreme amount of similarity, a very great similarity to prior product, and therefore would have very much smaller clinical trials needed, perhaps of immunogenicity.

Mr. WELCH. And that is an evaluation that you would feel confident, based on the information that you had at hand, that you could make?

Dr. WOODCOCK. Yes. FDA has a long history, as I said, of controlling the access to market after manufacturing changes for a very wide number of products for all pharmaceuticals on the market, and this is another example of that.

Mr. WELCH. I was going to ask another question, but you are starting to answer it. What scientific developments have allowed FDA to feel that confidence you are describing, that manufacturers of existing biologics can change cell lines, manufacturing facilities, and/or the fermentation processes without having it conduct those clinical trials?

Dr. WOODCOCK. Yes. And, as I said, sometimes they do and sometimes they don't. It really depends. The burden is on them, the manufacturer, to show through scientific data that the performance of the product after the change process is going to be the same as the performance of the product before the change.

Mr. WELCH. And are clinical trials always the most sensitive studies for detecting changes in safety or effectiveness due to process changes?

Dr. WOODCOCK. No. No, I think that is a common misconception. Clinical trials may be insensitive to certain types of changes, adverse effects, for example, that are rare or uncommon.

Mr. WELCH. Yes.

Dr. WOODCOCK. And we really need to use the scientific tool to assess the change in the product that is appropriate. It might be physical characterization or it might be a functional test. It might be evaluation of the purity of the product.

Mr. WELCH. Thank you. I yield the balance of my time.

Chairman WAXMAN. Thank you for yielding. You have another minute left on your time, so if the gentleman would permit I will take that minute if he will yield to me.

Dr. Woodcock, if FDA were given broad authority to require any studies necessary for approval of follow-on versions of PHS Act approved protein products, are you comfortable that the agency could use its discretion to ensure that only safe and effective products were made available to patients? I think you have answered that question several times, but let me just put it very clearly.

Dr. WOODCOCK. I think that FDA must do that. All right? We do not currently approve generic products unless they have absolutely met our standards and were follow-on products under 505(b)(2). We must maintain the confidence in our program and also our own scientific integrity.

Chairman WAXMAN. Based on your experience with the comparability guidance, can you give the committee a perspective on how often companies must do clinical outcome trials, not just PK or PD studies, to support a product or process change after approval of its BLA? Are large clinical outcome studies scientifically essential to support the approval 1 out of 10 post-approval product changes, 1 out of 20 post-approval changes, or 1 out of 50 changes?

Dr. WOODCOCK. I would say that the factor that is most important here is the magnitude of the change; however, it is probably more in the 1 in 50 range than the 1 in 10, or whatever. But don't forget there are many different types of changes that occur all the time to manufacturing processes. If you included all of those, then requiring clinical studies of outcomes would probably be quite rare.

Chairman WAXMAN. Thank you.

Mr. Bilbray.

Mr. BILBRAY. Mr. Chairman, I would like to yield my time to the gentleman from the Northwest Territory, but I would first like to clarify that, as a native Californian as opposed to Mr. Issa who is an immigrant, I was outraged at the concept of bringing a bottle of Merlot to this table and having it chilled. [Laughter.]

The only thing worse than that is to take it from the table and take it back to his office after he presented it.

But at this time I would like to yield to Mr. Burton.

Mr. BURTON. I thank the gentleman for yielding. I am from the Midwest, not the northwest.

Mr. BILBRAY. Well, the Northwest Territory.

Mr. BURTON. Ohio, the Northwest Territory. You are going back a long way.

First of all, let me preface my remarks by saying the pharmaceutical industry and FDA working together has created probably the highest quality of life in the history of mankind, and I appreciate that and I think everybody in America does. There are some questions, though, that I have to ask about the process.

You said it is a judgment call on whether or not this product comes to market. Who makes the judgment? Who makes the call?

Dr. WOODCOCK. The FDA.

Mr. BURTON. Don't they have advisory committees that review the process, review the product, review the results, and then they make a recommendation to the FDA?

Dr. WOODCOCK. Yes. Advisory committees are frequently utilized, particularly on clinical decisions. Here we are talking about scientific characterization of the product in a wide variety of ways. Most often, that is something that the FDA scientists do.

Mr. BURTON. But the FDA does have advisory committees for almost all of the products?

Dr. WOODCOCK. Yes.

Mr. BURTON. When I was chairman I asked—I don't believe it was you, but I asked one of your coworkers who was a leader at the FDA how many times has an advisory committee recommendation been turned down by the FDA.

Dr. WOODCOCK. You are asking me?

Mr. BURTON. Yes.

Dr. WOODCOCK. I don't know the answer to that.

Mr. BURTON. I will tell you what it was before. It was never. The advisory committee, I was told by the people who were doing the investigation for my committee when I was chairman, was that the advisory committee recommendations were always accepted.

Now, the other thing I would like to know is: the people on the advisory committee, do they file financial disclosure reports?

Dr. WOODCOCK. Yes, they do.

Mr. BURTON. We looked at some of the financial disclosure reports when I was holding hearings on this when I was chairman and we found that many of the people in the advisory committees did not file financial disclosure reports. And we found that some on the advisory committees had a conflict of interest. The RotoShield virus was one of those. The head of the advisory committee had an interest in a company that was going to make a RotoShield virus vaccine, which was put on the market at his advisory committee's recommendation, and FDA approved it based upon the recommendation. One or two children died and several people were injured and they pulled it off the market within 12 months.

I bring this up because this is a very important issue we are talking about today, and I would just like to ask that these advisory committees, when they make recommendation, that there is a thorough judgment made after the advisory committee makes its determination, and that the FDA does not always accept their results or their recommendations, and that there are complete financial disclosure reports.

The reason for that is pretty obvious. If a person is on an advisory committee and their recommendation is accepted and they have a financial interest in a pharmaceutical company that is going to manufacture a product like that or a like product, they are liable to have their judgment tainted just a little bit. It has happened in the past and I hope it doesn't happen in the future.

The cost of biotech drugs increased 17 percent from 2005 to 2006, and that was compared to 5.4 percent increase for traditional pharmaceuticals, which are much more expensive here than in some other countries, in most cases. Why was that increase so much? Do you know?

Dr. WOODCOCK. My understanding is that some of the new biotech products on the market that are very highly effective, you know, are very expensive to purchase, as some of the members already alluded to. But I don't have any complete analysis of this.

Mr. BURTON. I have a couple more questions, but I will wait.

Chairman WAXMAN. We will have another round.

Mr. BURTON. I will catch it next time.

Dr. WOODCOCK. May I?

Chairman WAXMAN. Yes.

Dr. WOODCOCK. The FDA has recently published new guidance on advisory committee conflicts of interest, and it lays out very explicit and transparent guidance on how people will be evaluated for their conflicts of interest.

Mr. BURTON. That is very good news. I appreciate hearing that. That is a great step in the right direction. Thank you.

Chairman WAXMAN. Thank you, Mr. Burton.

Mr. Davis.

Mr. DAVIS OF ILLINOIS. Thank you very much, Mr. Chairman.

Dr. Woodcock, I have always tried to understand—and if you could enlighten me it would be very helpful to me—the real difference between generic drugs and the brand name drugs. If they do essentially the same thing or if the level of effectiveness is essentially the same, why do we pay so much more for one as opposed to the other? I have never been able to, in my own mind, feel that I had a real understanding of that.

Dr. WOODCOCK. Well, if I may, if you look at the diagram—it is gone now, but there was a diagram of the molecule up there, a small molecule. We know exactly everything how that molecule is structured. We know everything about it.

And so what we do in the generic drug program is we require an exact copy of that molecule to be the generic drug and then we make sure that molecule gets into the body the exact same way that the innovator molecule gets into the body. So then we say if it does that it is going to have the same effect on the body because it is circulating around in the body the same way as the innovator drug. So that is what a generic drug is.

The problem with the proteins is it is very difficult to say we have the exact same molecule because it is such a complicated molecule.

Mr. DAVIS OF ILLINOIS. The effectiveness or the impact, are we saying that we would expect a different level of impact or effectiveness using one as opposed to the other?

Dr. WOODCOCK. For the generic drugs that FDA approves we expect the exact same performance. Now, that means the exact same good effects and the exact same side effects as the drug it is a copy of.

Mr. DAVIS OF ILLINOIS. Do you know then how the price or cost differential emerges or is determined?

Dr. WOODCOCK. Well, while the innovator drug is patent protected or protected by exclusivity, there are no other copies available to be prescribed. During that time the price is quite high. Once generic versions get in the market, the price of the various generic copies becomes only a fraction of what was charged by the innovator.

Mr. DAVIS OF ILLINOIS. Are you aware or familiar with any consumer studies that would indicate whether or not consumers have a greater level of confidence, for example, in the more popular pharmaceuticals than the generics?

Dr. WOODCOCK. Certainly the generics are not advertised and certainly there is some brand name loyalty that I have heard of. I have certainly talked to many, many consumers over my lifetime about this issue. There is some residual concern still about the generics and whether are they as good because they are not the brand name product; however, I think in the last 10 or 12 years of our generic drug program, confidence, both by the health professionals—the pharmacists, the doctors—as well as the consumers has really risen, and most people in this country are used to taking generic versions.

Mr. DAVIS OF ILLINOIS. And so then one could probably reasonably assume that marketing plays a great role in shaping our attitudes and thoughts about the drugs that we would most likely prefer using?

Dr. WOODCOCK. I can't comment on that directly, but that is one of the purposes of advertising.

Mr. DAVIS OF ILLINOIS. And so I would assume that it probably works fairly well and that it does, in fact, skew one's thinking. And if we are talking about having the most cost-effective health care, then it just seems to me that the more enlightened consumers become, that will probably have as much impact on cost effectiveness in health care as anything that we are going to regulate or anything that we are going to do.

I thank you very much for your answers.

Dr. WOODCOCK. At the request of Congress, we had an education program, outreach program, on the generic drug program. It has been very effective.

Mr. DAVIS OF ILLINOIS. Thank you. Thank you very much.

And thank you, Mr. Chairman. I yield back.

Chairman WAXMAN. Thank you, Mr. Davis.

Mr. Burton was using Mr. Bilbray's time, and he said he had a few more questions, so before we go to a second round I yield to you your first-round 5 minutes.

Mr. BURTON. Thank you. I just have a few more questions.

Dr. Woodcock, I think you have been very helpful, some of your answers today. I really appreciate that.

The pharmaceutical industry deserves to get some of their money back or all of their money back when they spend a lot of money on research and development, and that is why the patents are there, and then when it expires, of course, it can be a generic drug and they should have recovered their investment.

Are other countries working to develop these biotech drugs?

Dr. WOODCOCK. Yes. As was alluded to earlier, the European Union has published a directive and is implementing a program on what they call biosimilars. By that generally they mean biotech drugs.

Mr. BURTON. If they produce a biotech drug and there is a similar biotech drug that has been produced here in the United States, because of the differences, the scientific differences that you were talking about when we saw the slide a while ago, the FDA probably would not allow that drug to be imported into the United States until it was approved by the FDA, even though it did the same thing or pretty much the same thing?

Dr. WOODCOCK. Yes. The law doesn't allow drugs to be imported in the United States unless they are approved.

Mr. BURTON. Let me ask you one more question. If we had reimportation or importation of the pharmaceuticals that are approved by the FDA, would the prices of those pharmaceuticals be lower?

Dr. WOODCOCK. Again, this is beyond my area of expertise. I apologize.

Mr. BURTON. I will just followup by saying that everybody wants free enterprise to succeed and they want the pharmaceutical industry to make a lot of money so that they can do continued research, but when my first wife had cancer—and I have talked about this before—we went to have her chemotherapy and the tamoxifen that one woman was taking, she was complaining about the cost being about $300 a month, and another lady said I'm getting the same thing from Canada for $50 a month, so it was six times less.

There are a number of us in Congress that would like to see the FDA working with their counterparts in other countries and the pharmaceutical companies working with their counterparts in other countries and the governments of other countries to find out some way to level the playing field so that Americans are paying a comparable price for their pharmaceutical products as they do in other countries. It just doesn't seem fair to go to Germany or France or Spain or Canada and find that the very same product is being sold for much less, and Americans are paying actually a great deal more for the research and development and the advertising than is being paid elsewhere.

That is just a suggestion. I appreciate very much your candid answers.

I yield to the chairman.

Chairman WAXMAN. Thank you very much for yielding. The gentleman has a minute and a half, so I will be glad to take it.

If a statute were passed giving FDA broad authority to review abbreviated applications for follow-on proteins, and if companies were ready to begin submitting applications as soon as the statute became law, is it reasonable to assume that FDA would be able to begin reviewing those applications as soon as they were submitted, assuming, for the purpose of this question, that the statute did not require FDA to issue regulations or guidance as a prerequisite to the review of applications?

Dr. WOODCOCK. FDA is currently, as I said, reviewing applications and also inquiries from companies and so forth, providing guidance for drugs under the 505(b)(2) regimen. So we have the technical expertise to perform these functions.

Chairman WAXMAN. Thank you.

Mr. Hodes.

Mr. HODES. Thank you, Mr. Chairman.

Dr. Woodcock, I want to focus for a moment on the issue of comparability.

Dr. WOODCOCK. Yes.

Mr. HODES. It is my understanding that biologics as a group are so diverse and in some cases so incompletely understood that there is today no one-size-fits-all set of studies that can demonstrate comparability. Is that true?

Dr. WOODCOCK. Absolutely. Biologics, as opposed to biotech proteins, range from everything from gene therapy to cells, living cells of different types, to tissues—a huge range of different kind of products.

Mr. HODES. And am I correct that biopharmaceutical products often undergo changes after approval and that pre-change and post-change products will be comparable, as opposed to identical?

Dr. WOODCOCK. Yes. As we were discussing before, manufacturers need to continue to improve their process or they may need to open up new plants or increase the level of production, the scale of production. There are a lot of changes that have to be made. After each one of those changes, we must assess whether or not the performance of the product has changed.

Mr. HODES. And the FDA establishes boundaries and batches. Different batches have to fall within established boundaries for that product?

Dr. WOODCOCK. Yes. Any product, whether it is a small molecule or drug, has slight variations lot to lot in any kind of testing parameter that you would put on it, so the traditional approach is to establish boundaries within which a product can vary, but it can't go outside of those limits.

Mr. HODES. Now, just as the science is evolving on the manufacturing side— certainly from the FDA's standpoint techniques for assessing the structure and activity of biologics are evolving rapidly—and our understanding of biological structure and activity is improving all the time; is that correct?

Dr. WOODCOCK. That is correct.

Mr. HODES. If Congress were to tell the FDA what specific types of clinical data must always be required for approval of follow-on biologics based on today's science, could such clinical data requirements become obsolete?

Dr. WOODCOCK. Certainly, from my point of view, flexibility in enabling us to incorporate the new science into the regulatory process as that science evolves and becomes available is in the best interest of the public as well as the agency and the industry.

Mr. HODES. And if a follow-on statute required a clinical trial in every case, could it end up requiring perhaps unnecessary and therefore potentially unethical trials in the future?

Dr. WOODCOCK. Where trials aren't needed, it is, you know, of questionable ethics to repeat them. So use of human subjects for trials that are not needed or done simply to check a box on a regulatory requirement are not desirable.

Mr. HODES. Let me ask you a question about the EU system. The EU regulations, as I understand them—imperfectly, I might add—require post-market surveillance; is that correct?

Dr. WOODCOCK. I can't speak exactly. The Europeans have the ability to require post-marketing surveillance for any approved pharmaceutical.

Mr. HODES. Does the FDA currently have any requirements for post-market surveillance?

Dr. WOODCOCK. We very frequently request post-marketing studies be performed at the time of approval, and those are agreed to by the firms.

Mr. HODES. So it is the manufacturers who are conducting the post-market surveillance?

Dr. WOODCOCK. Yes.

Mr. HODES. The FDA relies on the manufacturers for that postmarket surveillance; the FDA doesn't do any of its own?

Dr. WOODCOCK. Right. The FDA conducts the adverse event reporting system, which is an adverse event reports from doctors and companies, and we do some limited studies, but in general we do not have the capacity to do post-marketing surveillance as you are describing.

Mr. HODES. Do you believe with biogenerics developing as rapidly as the field is developing, there should be expanded requirements for post-market surveillance?

Dr. WOODCOCK. All pharmaceuticals when they are approved for the first time have a fair amount of uncertainty still surrounding them about their performance, and particularly, as we have discussed already, any protein product that would be approved would continue to have questions about immunogenicity and perhaps other side effects that would probably need to continue to be looked at in the post-marketing period.

Mr. HODES. Can the FDA require post-marketing studies?

Dr. WOODCOCK. What we do is say to the company: you need to agree to conduct this study, and if you do then that is part of the approval the company agrees to do.

Mr. HODES. So, if I understand your answer, the answer is yes, the FDA does have the authority to require post-market studies? Dr. WOODCOCK. At the time of approval.

Mr. HODES. And what proportion of post-market studies that you require are completed?

Dr. WOODCOCK. That is a complicated question. There are many different types of studies that are requested, and some of them go on a long time, so there isn't a really high proportion. I don't know the exact number, because it depends on what analysis you are doing, but many of these studies are not completed.

Mr. HODES. And if you were the last word on this, thinking about where the science is going with biogenerics, do you see a need for increased requirements for post-market studies of these biogenerics, none of which will ever be identical, either in batch or in actual structure, to the original?

Dr. WOODCOCK. I believe it would be likely in many cases, but, as I said, this is going to be case-by-case because of all the differences in the different products.

In many cases FDA would need to have post-marketing surveillance or post-marketing studies done to resolve remaining uncertainties.

Mr. HODES. And, last question, does the FDA have an enforcement mechanism to require completion of any post-marketing studies that you have required of the manufacturers?

Dr. WOODCOCK. We can publicize the fact that the studies have not been done, and we could take the drug off the market.

Mr. HODES. So the enforcement mechanism is the possible removal of the drug from the market for lack of completion?

Dr. WOODCOCK. Yes.

Mr. HODES. Has that ever been done?

Dr. WOODCOCK. Not to my knowledge.

Mr. HODES. Thank you.

I yield back. Thank you, Mr. Chairman.

Chairman WAXMAN. Thank you. That is called the guillotine, except it is never used.

Dr. Woodcock, I understand that it is quite a bit more complicated to establish interchangeability of two protein products than to establish their comparable safety and effectiveness. Would it be possible to demonstrate that a copy of a well-understood protein is interchangeable with the brand name drug if there are no limits on what studies can be required?

Dr. WOODCOCK. We believe so. The situation in health care right now is that products that are interchangeable, they may be repeatedly switched back and forth. All right? And where you have a situation where you have a number of similar products on the market, the same indication, and they are very similar, it might be that they can be switched back and forth among one another multiple times for a given patient, depending on the plan and who they contract with and so on. In that situation either the innovator product could cause antibodies to the follow-on product or vice versa. We think we would have to test that in people to make sure, but we think it would be feasible to do those tests.

Chairman WAXMAN. Is our understanding of protein structure and activity likely to evolve in a way that will make it possible to establish interchangeability in the foreseeable future, at least for some of these proteins, that may not be obvious at the present time?

Dr. WOODCOCK. It may not be the protein, itself, that causes the immune response, but it could be different contaminants that are co-purified from the cell line or during the manufacturing process, or it can be changes that happen late in manufacturing or during storage or so forth, so it is really a very complicated situation.

Chairman WAXMAN. For very simple, well-understood proteins, what kinds of studies might be required to establish interchangeability?

Dr. WOODCOCK. Well, a study that actually performs that activity, which changes the patient back and forth from one version of the product to the next and follows the immune response.

Chairman WAXMAN. Would that be a difficult study?

Dr. WOODCOCK. No. In some cases there might be ethical issues that we would have to address very carefully. We would not want to set any patient up for harm.

Chairman WAXMAN. Might the study requirements lessen over time as the molecules are better understood?

Dr. WOODCOCK. Yes.

Chairman WAXMAN. Do you think that the FDA would ever declare a copy of a biotech drug regulated under Hatch-Waxman to be interchangeable if the agency had doubts about whether it could be safely substituted for the brand name product?

Dr. WOODCOCK. No. I mean, we believe that our finding of an A rating of interchangeability is our word. We are saying that scientifically we believe those products would be interchangeable, and we would not do that unless we believed that were the case and it was substantiated with scientific data.

Chairman WAXMAN. Do you think that the FDA could be trusted to make appropriate interchangeability determinations for protein products if the agency were given statutory authority to approve copies of biologics under the PHS Act?

Dr. WOODCOCK. I believe that the FDA can be trusted to carry out its mandate from Congress, whatever that might be.

Chairman WAXMAN. And if we gave you an additional mandate, you feel you would be able to live up to it?

Dr. WOODCOCK. Yes. I believe we have scientific expertise. As we have already discussed, we have been managing manufacturing changes for all pharmaceuticals on the market for a very long time.

Chairman WAXMAN. Thank you.

Let me see if any Member wishes additional time for questions?

[No response.]

Chairman WAXMAN. If not, let me thank you very much for your presentation and your willingness to answer these questions. I think it has been very helpful for us in our understanding of this issue. Thank you very much.

Dr. WOODCOCK. Thank you.

Chairman WAXMAN. The Chair would like to now call forward our second panel.

Dr. Geoffrey Allan is the president, CEO, and chairman of the Board of Insmed Incorporated located in Richmond, VA. Insmed is a biopharmaceutical company focused on the development and commercialization of drugs for the treatment of metabolic diseases and endocrine disorders with unmet medical needs.

Dr. Theresa L. Gerrard is now the president of TLG Consulting, Inc., where she assists pharmaceutical and biotechnology companies in product development and regulatory strategy. Prior to that she spent 11 years as a Division Director in FDA's Center for Biologics Evaluation and Research, and she has also previously served as director of development for Amgen.

Dr. Bill Schwieterman is a physician and scientist by training who now acts as an industry consultant to major biotech pharmaceutical companies on product clinical development issues. Dr. Schwieterman started his career at NIH and subsequently moved to FDA, where he worked for 10 years and served as the Chief of Immunology and Infectious Disease Branch within FDA's Center for Biologics Evaluation and Research.

Inger Mollerup has been the vice president for regulatory affairs at Nova Nordisk A/S since 2004. Nova Nordisk is a pharmaceutical company which focuses on diabetes care, as well as hemostasis management, growth hormone therapy, and hormone replacement therapy.

Dr. Ganesh Venkataraman is co-founder and senior vice president of research at Momenta Pharmaceuticals. Momenta Pharmaceuticals, Inc., is a biotechnology company located in Cambridge, MA focused on the treatment of disease through an understanding of sugars and complex biomolecules.

We are pleased to welcome all of you to our hearing today. We appreciate your being here.

It is the custom of this committee to put all witnesses under oath. You are not being singled out. I would like to ask you to please stand and raise your right hands.

[Witnesses sworn.]

Chairman WAXMAN. The record will reflect that each member answered in the affirmative.

We will make your prepared statements part of the record in its entirety. We would like to ask, if you would, to try to limit the oral presentation to around 5 minutes.

Why don't we start with Dr. Allan, and then we will move right down the line. You see we do have a timer. Dr. Allen.

STATEMENTS OF GEOFFREY ALLEN, PH.D, PRESIDENT, CHIEF EXECUTIVE OFFICER, CHAIRMAN OF THE BOARD, INSMED INC.; THERESA LEE GERRARD, PH.D, PRESIDENT, TLG CONSULTING, INC. (BIOPHARMACEUTICAL CONSULTANTS FORMERLY WITH AMGEN AND FDA'S CENTER FOR BIOLOGICS); BILL SCHWIETERMAN, M.D., PRESIDENT, TEKGENICS CORP. (BIOPHARMACEUTICAL CONSULTANTS FORMERLY WITH FDA'S CENTER FOR BIOLOGICS); INGER MOLLERUP, VICE PRESIDENT FOR REGULATORY AFFAIRS, NOVA NORDISK A/S; AND GANESH VENKATARAMAN, PH.D, SENIOR VICE PRESIDENT, RESEARCH, MOMENTA PHARMACEUTICALS, INC.

Statement of Geoffrey Allan

Mr. ALLAN. Good morning, Chairman Waxman, Ranking Member Davis, and members of the Oversight and Government Reform Committee. I am delighted to have the opportunity to testify before your committee. The focus of my discussion will be the role of small, innovative biotechnology companies in the current debate regarding the development of a regulatory pathway for approving biogeneric drugs.

My name is Geoffrey Allan, and I currently serve as the chief executive officer of Insmed, Inc. Insmed is a small biotechnology company focused on the development and commercialization of drugs for the treatment of metabolic and endocrine disorders where there are clear unmet medical needs.

We received FDA approval for our lead product, IPLEX, at the end of 2005. IPLEX is a therapeutic protein which is approved for the treatment of children suffering from a rare growth disorder. We are currently continuing to develop IPLEX for several major medical illnesses such as myotonic muscular dystrophy and medical complications associated with HIV infection.

I am here today to talk about biogeneric drug development and the regulatory path forward. I believe our experience with IPLEX is very illustrative of the scientific and technical issues confronting biogeneric drug developers, issues such as comparability testing and the nature and extent of clinical trials needed to support characterization of a generic biologic. Our experience tells us that these issues can be addressed using sound, readily available scientific approach.

Insmed has developed significant intellectual capital focused toward protein characterization and purification. We have invested in building a facility required to manufacture quality proteins. The biogenerics business is a business in which we would like to specialize. The combination of our proprietary protein platform with a biogeneric protein platform meets our goal to sustain innovation, along with the ability to provide safe and affordable drugs to address a growing economic issue.

It is my belief that there are a number of my colleagues in similarsized companies that are also interested in providing the scientific expertise to meet the challenges of producing biogenerics. I believe that I am representing the interests of many smaller biotechnology companies and large contract manufacturing companies. I believe H.R. 1038 provides for a fair balance between reward and innovation in creating a timely approval pathway in commercialization of biogenerics in the marketplace; therefore, passing this bill would be a positive step for the biotech industry and continue to fuel the cycle of innovation.

As the chief executive officer of a small biotechnology company, I hope my testimony will provide a different perspective on this important issue and bring to light some of the important reasons why this bill is the correct model to create a robust, competitive, and innovation biopharmaceutical marketplace.

IPLEX is a recombinant protein product. In fact, it is a combination of two different recombinant protein molecules. It is a relatively large molecule, larger than insulin, growth hormone, the interferons, and Epogen, and certainly no less complex in its structural characteristics. As a new drug, along with the demonstration of safety and efficacy in the target population, structural characterization of the protein and the development of a quality manufacturing process was our central focus during the development of the product.

During the course of the development of this product, we modified the manufacturing process several times. We changed cell lines. We changed purification procedures. We changed raw material sources. And on more than one occasion we changed the facilities where this product was manufactured. At all times, good analytical methodology was the bedrock of our comparability testing to ensure that we produced a consistent, highly purified protein.

Analytical methodology to allow structural characterization of proteins has evolved enormously over the years. It is sophisticated and has exquisite sensitivity. For example, we use a battery of sensitive and analytical tests. More than 10 of these tests are used, one of which is a technology called mass spectroscopy. This technique has such high resolution that on certain molecules we can detect changes as small as a single proton within the molecule. This is essentially not a crude science.

During the development of IPLEX we worked closely with the FDA. They clearly used their discretion to decide what tests we needed to support our scientific approach as we made changes to our manufacturing processes. Their recommendations were rational and certainly not onerous. On the occasion that we changed the site of manufacture of the drug, moving our process from a U.K. facility to our own facility in Colorado, we conducted a simple pharmacokinetic study in human volunteers to establish the equivalence of the products after the facility change. We established very quickly, within 1 month, that the amount of drug in the bloodstream was consistent, regardless of where the drug was manufactured.

IPLEX was being developed for use in children, and as such both we and the FDA knew that safety at all times was paramount and was certainly never jeopardized. For example, FDA was concerned that immunogenicity of the product could vary as we changed the process. We established surveillance procedures to address this issue, and we continue to monitor for signs of immunogenicity today.

I have only given you a very brief overview of the type of scientific and technical issues we had to address in the development of this product, IPLEX; however, these issues are at the heart of what a biogeneric manufacturer would have to confront. The science has reached a level of sophistication to make this endeavor entirely possible. All we need now is the regulatory go-ahead.

The proposal introduced by Chairman Waxman is extremely appealing as a next step in stimulating competition in order to address an ever-increasing economic problem facing our health care system. Based on our company's experience with the FDA during the approval process of IPLEX, I am confident that this legislation is based on sound science and progressive insight into where the market should be in the coming years.

Once again, thank you for this unique and important opportunity to share my experience and views. I look forward to your questions.

[The prepared statement of Mr. Allan follows:]

Chairman WAXMAN. Thank you very much, Dr. Allan.

Dr. Gerrard.

Statement of Theresa Gerrard

Ms. GERRARD. Good morning, Chairman Waxman, Ranking Member Davis, and members of the committee. My name is Theresa Gerrard. Thank you for allowing me the opportunity to testify this morning on the importance of establishing a science-based, abbreviated approval pathway for biogenerics.

From 1984 to 1995 I was with the FDA and was a Division Director with responsibility for IND and BLA review of hundreds of biotech products. I chaired licensing committees for Amgen's Neupogen, Genentech's Actimmune, and was involved in the review of beta Interferon from Chiron and Biogen.

After leaving FDA, I was director of development for Amgen in Boulder, CO, where I had oversight of development of several biotech products. For the past 9 years I have worked as a consultant, where I have worked with many companies, primarily brand biotech companies.

The purity of biotech products and the sophistication of analytical testing that exists today allowed the production of safe biotech drugs. Analytical testing consists of multiple sophisticated tests that are used to assess the physical, chemical, and biological characteristics of the product. Many more tests are used to assess a biologic than are typically used to assess a drug, because biotech products are more complex than drugs.

These tests set the product specifications or goalposts, if you will, for every batch of biotech product that must fall between these goalposts. This is because no two batches of biotech products are identical. There are always minor variations.

The advances in analytical characterization for well-characterized biologics allowed FDA to develop scientific policy officers on comparability in the early 1990's. This gave brand manufacturers the ability to change the manufacturing processes without the need for redoing the original clinical outcome trials if the product generated by the new process was shown to be comparable to product made by the old process.

Now, when we speak of biologic, the focus is on comparability. Why? Because no two batches of biologic product, whether brand name or generic, will ever be identical. Therefore, biologics are and should always be discussed in the context of comparability. Yes, small changes in manufacturing could have an impact on the final product, but we have known this for more than a decade and can detect these changes.

For the past 15 years, FDA has gained substantial experience and expertise in assessing manufacturing changes and comparability data for a large number of protein products. The underlying scientific principles that have guided comparability policy are still valid and can, and should be adopted for the generic bio pharmaceuticals. Why? Because the types of post-approval brand product changes are reflective of the issues biotech and generic companies will face in bringing generic biotech products to the market.

The primary premise of comparability is that analytical testing is the most sensitive method to detect differences between two products. Clinical trials are rather insensitive in detecting product differences because the variation among people and their responses to a biopharmaceutical do not allow one to detect subtle product differences. Analytical testing, by itself, will not be sufficient in every case to demonstrate that a generic will have the same safety and efficacy as the brand name biotech product. In those cases, FDA can require additional data such as animal studies, human pharmacokinetic studies, or even clinical trials. There is not a onesize-fits-all model, but FDA can determine the amount of data needed based on the complexity of the product, the history of the clinical use, and the extent of analytical characterization to determine its comparability with the brand name product.

Before concluding, the question of immunogenicity has been raised in the discussion of both brand name and generic biopharmaceuticals, and I would like to take a moment to just briefly touch on this topic.

Immunogenicity means the body generates antibodies to a specific foreign substance, such as bacteria, and it is a normal response in keeping people healthy. People routinely make antibodies to many different substances and experience no negative effects. Some biologics can cause people to generate antibodies which are specific to that product, but most will not have any affect on safety or efficacy. For some to imply that immunogenicity reactions are always harmful is just plain incorrect.

FDA can assess the risk for immunogenicity when it reviews the products for purity, safety, and overall quality and can request additional clinical data when necessary. While immunogenicity is an important consideration for biogenerics, it is certainly not a hurdle to their development.

Mr. Chairman, the science exists for a creation of a clear, efficient, abbreviated biogeneric approval pathway. Analytical tests, combined with additional data when needed, would ensure the safety and efficacy of generic biopharmaceuticals.

Thank you.

[The prepared statement of Ms. Gerrard follows:]

Chairman WAXMAN. Thank you very much, Dr. Gerrard.

Dr. Schwieterman.

Statement of William Schwieterman

Dr. SCHWIETERMAN. Good morning, Chairman Waxman and members of the Committee on Oversight and Government Reform.

My name is Dr. William Schwieterman. I thank you for the opportunity to appear before the committee today and present the scientific and clinical perspective on the issue of biogenerics.

One of the most disturbing experiences for a physician is to know that a treatment is available to help your patient, but the cost may simply be beyond what your patient can afford. For this reason, I deeply share your goal, Congressman Waxman, of creating a sound, scientifically based approval pathway for biogenerics. And, given that I also had the privilege of working at FDA in the area of biotechnology for 10 years, I know that your goal can and should be achieved.

I come before you today wearing three hats: as a physician, as a scientist, and as a former FDA reviewer. From this vantage point I would like to make the following critical points to the committee.

First, with today's scientific advancements and technologies, we can assure the safety and efficacy of biogenerics.

Second, the supporting science for this is not new. It has existed for over a decade.

Third, the issues raised in post-approval brand changes are reflective of the issues that are raised in the field of biogenerics. As such, the same science that determines comparability for the brand tech industry can also be adopted to ensure the safety and efficacy of complaint and interchangeable biogenerics.

Having worked extensively with agency physicians and scientists, it is clear to me that there is just one agency safety standard, and that standard has been and will continue to be applied in the review and approval of each and every biologic, whether it be a brand name or a generic.

The standards and science used for current biopharmaceuticals are informative to us with respect to biogenerics. A critical but not often publicized fact in the biopharmaceutical industry is that FDA does not require brand name companies to perform large clinical outcome studies to retest the product generated by new manufacturing processes. This is because such an approach would not only be infeasible, but, more importantly, would ignore the utility of existing sophisticated scientific analytic tools and techniques for this purpose.

Let me briefly summarize what happens in these instances. FDA starts with an assessment of extensive analytical comparability data. With these data, and keeping in mind the nature of the drug, the tests used, and the disease being studied, FDA decides how to proceed. The agency can give a thumbs-up or a thumbs-down regarding each post-approval brand manufacture change and, if thumbs-up, have that change be supported by the analytic data, alone. The analytic data, coupled with pharmacokinetic and/or pharmacodynamic studies or the analytic data—the studies just mentioned—plus data from a large clinical outcome study.

As you already have heard, the vast majority of brand name manufacturing changes need no further studies when data from analytic tests show the products to be comparable. For a small number of brand name products that show small differences in these analytic tests following manufacturing changes, FDA may require additional analytic tests and pharmacokinetic or pharmacodynamic tests to be conducted in animals or humans.

These later studies, PKBPD studies, are clinical studies in the sense that they are conducted in patients in the clinic, but they are not the large clinical outcome studies commonly used to determine the product's ultimate clinical effects.

These pharmacokinetic and pharmacodynamic studies almost always involve fewer than 100 patients, and in general last weeks, not many months.

Rarely after a brand name manufacturing change does the FDA require that a brand name company take the last step, repeating a full-scale clinical outcome study. Such studies are not usually necessary because the variability and ''noise'' involved in most clinical outcome studies make them inefficient for determining comparability between agents. In fact, of all the hundreds of brand name biologic product changes, the vast majority were approved without large clinical outcome trials.

In sum, FDA's scientists and physicians routinely make comparability determinations, since manufacturing changes occur throughout the brand name biologic product development and life cycle. The comparability algorithm has existed for over a decade to allow brand name biologic manufacturers to change and improve their manufacturing processes.

In closing, I want to emphasize to the committee again that the science of comparability is not a new one, but rather an old one used by the agency and the brand name industry for more than a decade to determine comparability.

Chairman Waxman, the Access to Life-Saving Medicines Act will give FDA the authority and the flexibility it needs to ensure the safety and efficacy of biogenerics. I commend you for adopting the same scientific principles, processes, and procedures that exist for the brand name biologic industry when making post-approval manufacturing product changes to the biogeneric sector.

My mission as a physician reviewer at FDA, and that of all my colleagues, then and now, is to protect the public by ensuring the safety of the supply of biopharmaceuticals. No one's interests is served if safety is not viewed as paramount.

Thank you very much.

[The prepared statement of Dr. Schwieterman follows:]

Chairman WAXMAN. Thank you very much, Dr. Schwieterman.

Ms. Mollerup.

Statement of Inger Mollerup

Ms. MOLLERUP. Chairman Waxman, Ranking Member Davis, members of the committee, thank you for inviting me to testify today. My name is Inger Mollerup. I am vice president for regulatory affairs of Nova Nordisk, a company with an 80-year history of producing insulin and other proteins.

I am a scientist, not a lawyer, and as such have for the last 30 years been engaged in the design of manufacturing processes and development programs for numerous recombinant proteins. In 2005 I represented the drug before the European Medicines Agency [EMEA], discussing the insulin follow-on guidance, and I also presented to the World Health Organization's INN Committee on issues related to naming of all therapeutic proteins, including follow-ons.

Nova Nordisk believes that any pathway for follow-on biologics must be, first and foremost, constructed to protect patient safety, be rooted in the best science, preserve innovation, and respect proprietary information.

Three major points from my testimony today are: first, that characterization does not tell the whole story; second, that pre-clinical and laboratory tests are not sufficient to determine immunogenicity and other important safety parameters; and, third, that current science does not support interchangeability.

First, characterization does not tell the whole story. Any pathway must fully address the patient safety considerations of medicines that are similar to or comparable to instead of the same as the reference product. Given that proposals currently before Congress go far beyond the science in an effort to deem products having minor differences in immuno-acid sequence as highly similar, I share with you an experience we had at Nova Nordisk as we were developing a fast-acting insulin analog wherein two potential candidates with one amino acid difference were tested.

All candidates were put into an extensive chemical preclinical and clinical program. The candidate taken to market had only one change to the immuno acid sequence from human insulin, resulting in an analog with significantly shorter timing of action than human insulin and a unique safety profile.

An earlier candidate, which had also one amino acid substitution, showed a positive effect on the timing of action, but in full preclinical animal toxicology studies this dark candidate significantly elevated tumor potential in rats. Development of this candidate was immediately discontinued.

Even though both analogs were fully characterized, an animal study was required to demonstrate that this seemingly minor difference had enormous consequences for important safety characteristics. Minor differences can have major safety consequences.

Second, pre-clinical and laboratory tests are not sufficient to determine immunogenicity and other important safety parameters. Human clinical immunogenicity data must be required, and we have numerous examples illustrating its vital importance.

While developing a complete new process for our insulin analog, we discussed this program with the FDA. FDA stated the no general safety threshold could be applied for new impurities. Even one as low as 0.1 percent was not acceptable because proteins can be immunogenic at very low concentrations, and it is not known when low is low enough. Immunogenicity data from an appropriate clinical study was, therefore, necessary and included in our submission.

Third, current science does not support interchangeability. Based on today's science, a follow-on biologic cannot be determined to be the same as a innovator drug. For this reason and because of the potential difference in immunogenicity and other drug-specific adverse events, follow-on biologic products must not be allowed to be interchangeable. The treating physician must at all times be involved in the decision to change from one product to another.

Interchangeability is also not part of the EMEA approval, and Europe has the further requirement that these products are clearly identified to support post-market monitoring.

Nova Nordisk believes that any pathway for follow-on biologics must be, first and foremost, constructed to protect patient safety, be rooted in the best science, preserve innovation, and respect proprietary information.

Thank you for the opportunity to speak here today. Nova Nordisk is ready to assist Congress as this issue moves forward.

[The prepared statement of Ms. Mollerup follows:]

Chairman WAXMAN. Thank you very much, Ms. Mollerup.

Dr. Venkataraman, we are pleased to have you with us.

Statement of Ganesh Venkataraman

Mr. VENKATARAMAN. Good morning, Chairman Waxman and members of the committee. I want to thank you for the invitation and opportunity to present to you this morning on this very important topic to our industry and for the general public.

I am Ganesh Venkataraman, co-founder and senior vice president of research at Momenta Pharmaceuticals. I am pleased to come before you today to discuss the scientific issues behind the need to create an abbreviated regulatory approval process for generic biologics, which are defined as follow-on protein products in Dr. Woodcock's testimony.

The terms that I use are also defined in the written testimony that we are submitting for the record.

Mr. Chairman, I am a chemical engineer by training, with specific expertise in bioprocess engineering, protein structure characterization, and analytic and quantitative methods for categorizing complex mixtures. While at MIT I, with Dr. Sasisekharan and Dr. Langer developed novel analytic technology that enables characterization of complex mixtures. With this platform and co-science and leadership at MIT, we founded Momenta. We develop novel drugs and generic versions of complex products. We use cutting edge science to develop affordable and safe generic versions of these products.

Momenta has a strong interest in ensuring that Congress acts this year. We believe our company's experience demonstrates that the science is available today and continues to evolve to enable generic versions of complex mixture drugs.

In my written testimony I focused on five major issues that I will briefly discuss today.

First point, complex biologics can be totally characterized. Not all biologic products are the same, so when we discuss the characterization challenges we must keep in mind the continuum of complexity. Analytic technologies are here today to characterize the less-complex biologics, and approaches like ours and others are actively being developed for those that are more complex.

In my testimony I highlight how our testimony is applied to heparins. While heparins are not biologics, it validates how complex mixtures can be characterized.

The second point is: with such product characterization, generic companies will be able to design and control the manufacturing process to reproducibly make biologic drugs with the same quality as the branded companies. The manufacturing process for biologic drugs does not occur in a random or uncontrolled system. The living cells are highly specialized systems which, in a very careful and controlled manner, produce a final product.

Scientific advances in analytical technologies available to the generic as well as the branded industries allow one to link process parameters to the final product. It is possible and absolutely critical that generic companies build and maintain the same level of process knowledge.

Point three: clinical studies, ranging from small-scale PK to clinical outcome studies, should be used to address any residual uncertainty answering relevant scientific questions. Traditional empirical or full-scale clinical trials must not be a requirement for approval in all cases. While the FDA may require full-scale trials for approval of some biologics, others that have an increased level of characterization data should require significantly reduced clinical testing.

We believe FDA is well equipped to work with applicants to determine the degree of testing necessary and define the characterization and trial requirements.

Point four: biologic drugs can be designed to be interchangeable. Interchangeability is an important public health objective and products need to be designed and proved to be interchangeable. It is well within the reach in the near term for a number of products. This can be done through total characterization and/or through a proper combination of characterization and clinical trials.

Point five: patient safety and product quality will not be jeopardized. We should hold the entire industry, branded and generic, alike, to the highest scientific standards, and allow the expertise of FDA's scientific staff, which will approve and oversee the marketing of innovator and generic biologics.

In closing, Mr. Chairman, there is an opportunity to drive continued scientific innovation by creating a forward-looking, regulated system which balances the respective roles that characterization and clinical data should play. FDA has to be given the opportunity to make the decisions on comparability, which is interchangeability based, on the science presented to them. If legislation does not allow for such a pathway today, scientific innovation from technology companies like ours and many others will be stifled, and access to more-affordable choices would be denied.

I hope that my perspectives will be instructive to this debate. I am confident that these efforts under your leadership will be a key contributor to increasing access to safe, effective, and affordable medications to patients in need.

I thank you again for the opportunity to submit testimony. I look forward to answering any questions.

[The prepared statement of Mr. Venkataraman follows:]

Chairman WAXMAN. Thank you very much, Dr. Venkataraman.

To begin the questioning, the Chair recognizes Mr. Burton.

Mr. BURTON. I thank the Chair for recognizing me. I have to go put a pharmaceutical in my eye at the hospital, so I can attest to the necessity for those products.

Mr. Chairman, I am not sure this question should be directed to the panel. It may be directed at you. From everything I have seen, there can be a minor difference in a biological product, and if the pharmaceutical company that created the product in the first place has to give a generic company the information before their patent expires, it seems to me, because of the minor difference that could be created by the generic company, they could apply for a license well before the patent runs out from the original producer. If that were the case, the scientific research being paid for by the original company, the pharmaceutical company that developed the product, could lose its investment after they have created something that is going to be beneficial to everybody.

So my question is: has that been checked out legally and whether or not the originating company can be protected for the duration of their patent?

Chairman WAXMAN. Perhaps we can let one of the panelists answer it, but it seems to me it becomes a patent question. If the originator of the product has a patent over that product, a minor variation, as you seem to describe it, would not be permitted as a competitor, if it is basically the same product.

Mr. BURTON. I think the bill has a great deal of merit.

Chairman WAXMAN. This is, of course, by the way, what we do right now with generics and brand name drugs. We allow generics to compete after the patent is over. If there is a new innovation in it or a minor difference, then the FDA would have to decide if it is, in fact, a generic.

Mr. BURTON. I understand that. I like the bill. That is one thing I would like to check out. Thank you, and thank you for yielding.

Chairman WAXMAN. Thank you very much.

The Chair recognizes himself.

Let me address this question to Dr. Gerrard and Dr. Schwieterman. As you testified, for over 10 years the FDA has allowed brand name manufactures of biotech drugs to make changes in the process by which they manufacture their products, but without repeating the original safety and effectiveness trials. This policy seems to me to undercut the brand name industry argument that changes in manufacturing processes can affect safety and effectiveness in ways that could only be assessed through clinical trials. In your judgment and experience, does permitting companies to make significant manufacturing changes under a comparability protocol, but without repeating clinical trials, adequately protect patients from unsafe or ineffective products?

Ms. GERRARD. I think, as both Dr. Woodcock and Dr. Schwieterman have said, FDA only has one standard for safety andefficacy, so when FDA makes the decision that, after a manufacturing change, that the product is comparable, they have decided that it is going to have the same safety and efficacy as the brand name product. What we are saying is some of those same principles apply to the development of generic biotech products.

Chairman WAXMAN. Yes.

Mr. SCHWIETERMAN. Yes, let me just add to that. The FDA is a science-based organization. It is filled with scientists. It is filled with physician reviewers. It is filled with people who are expert in data analysis and interpretation. Your question really is adking if the science there to allow in some cases for the absence of clinical trials, and I would say yes, it is there, but you would have to look at the data, you would have to look at the techniques, you would have to look at the actual agent under discussion. You take things on a case-by-case basis, based upon the science and the data, and then make that determination.

Chairman WAXMAN. Are there many examples of products approved under comparability protocols that turned out to have unpredicted safety or effectiveness problems that were only discovered after marketing?

Mr. SCHWIETERMAN. There are none in the United States where there were major changes in post-marketing that caused this. We all know the example of Eprex, which occurred post-marketing in Europe. The patients developed PRCA. But the agency and the biotechnology industry and biopharmaceutical industry in this country has been amazingly good at protecting the public this way.

Chairman WAXMAN. Does the scientific rationale underlying comparability protocols and FDA's 10 years of experience implementing it provide evidence that an abbreviated application process for follow-on proteins and biogenerics based on established comparability principles could adequately protect patients from unsafe or ineffective products? Dr. Gerrard.

Ms. GERRARD. I think the comparability policies have been enormously successful from FDA's point, and the American public has benefited, as well. Brand name companies have been able to make manufacturing changes and improve their product without the need to redo clinical trials.

I think we can apply some of those same principles in extending it one step further to generic biotech products.

Mr. SCHWIETERMAN. I would just like to add that I think the rationale is, in fact, one that can be used, coupled with the data, coupled with the case-by-case to develop a safe and effective biogeneric use of the principles we outlined.

Chairman WAXMAN. Dr. Schwieterman, Ms. Mollerup testified that immunogenicity can arise so unpredictably from changes in biologics that a follow-on biologic will always require a clinical trial to assess immunogenicity. When a brand name company uses the FDA's comparability guidance to make changes to its existing biologic products, are clinical trials always required to demonstrate that no new immunogenicity concerns have arisen?

Mr. SCHWIETERMAN. Always is an absolute, and absolutes are only things that can be supported by the data. FDA is a scientific organization, and I would say no. In every instance ought there be a clinical trial for immunogenicity? No. It would depend upon the nature of the case. It would depend on the data that are there. And I think there are ways and methods for sure beyond clinical trials to determine immunogenicity. In fact, clinical trials, themselves, have limitations in this regard, as they do with other infrequent safety AEs.

Chairman WAXMAN. Should there be more concern about immunogenicity for follow-on proteins than for brand name proteins?

Mr. SCHWIETERMAN. I don't think there should be more or less concern about immunogenicity. I think that the safety of all agents, particularly biogenerics and biopharmaceuticals in this country is a critical issue for the FDA. I think that the same standards, the same kinds of oversight, the same considerations for biogenerics ought to apply for them as they do for present-day biopharmaceuticals.

Chairman WAXMAN. Let me ask a question of Dr. Venkataraman and Dr. Allan. A number of companies have expressed doubts about whether copies of biotech drugs can be made safely. They have suggested that the manufacturing process for producing these drugs is so complex that new companies will not understand biologics manufacturing well enough to produce safe versions of these products. Isn't it true that there are a number of companies who already make brand name biotech drugs, either for themselves or on contract for other companies, who would be likely to want to make copies for biotech drugs if there were a legal pathway?

Mr. ALLAN. I believe there are contract manufacturing organizations that do make branded products, either at the research level, the development stage level, or even at the commercial level.

Chairman WAXMAN. Yes.

Mr. VENKATARAMAN. I would like to add I think the brand name manufacturers sometimes have made the process to be a black box. I think the science is there now to be able to go back and decouple product and relationship to the process so that you could use a different cell line and come up with a different process that would ultimately provide you the same end product. Provided you couple that with the characterization of looking at process-related impurities and end product, you could get there to the same level of being in a brand name manufacturer.

Chairman WAXMAN. Thank you very much.

Mr. Davis.

Mr. DAVIS OF VIRGINIA. Thank you, Mr. Waxman.

Ms. Mollerup, let me start with you. The generic system we created for pharmaceutical drugs in 1984, which bears Mr. Waxman's name, balanced and abbreviated approval systems for generic drugs with patent restoration and new exclusivity for innovators. Doesn't such a critical balance continue to stimulate the development of new cures for drugs, having that balance?

Ms. MOLLERUP. In my mind it is important that we keep the balance that will still foster innovation, and as this process goes forward toward defining a legislative and regulatory system, that is acknowledged, because you would still want new drugs to come on the market in this country.

Mr. DAVIS OF VIRGINIA. What kind of impact would a system that fails to assure safety or sustain innovator intellectual property rights have on innovation?

Ms. MOLLERUP. A system that would fail to protect safety I think would be detrimental for both innovation and follow-on manufactures, and obviously first and foremost for public health. I think it is very important, as Congress moves forward, that the pathway you are moving toward is really constructed to protect patient safety and be rooted in the best science, and there is a lot of strong and good science available for this.

Mr. DAVIS OF VIRGINIA. The FDA stated in its testimony that demonstrating the similarity of a follow-on protein product to a reference product is more complex and would require new data. I guess my question is: does this mean FDA should require clinical safety data for follow-on biologics, or do you think there are cases where they could make the determination it wouldn't?

Ms. MOLLERUP. Based on my experience with those complete second-generation processes that we have developed and are developing at Nova Nordisk, these require immunogenicity data in all cases for the simpler ones like insulin, described in my testimony. Besides that, PKPD was required to assess both pharmacokinetics and efficacy for a more complex one like a co-correlation factor, substantial clinical data will be required, as well as immunogenicity.

So, based on the experience that we have with processes that have less substantial changes than follow-ons, from my standpoint, where the science is today, immunogenicity trials will always be required.

Mr. DAVIS OF VIRGINIA. Thank you.

Let me ask Dr. Venkataraman and Dr. Allan, you are both from small biotech companies. FDA stated in their testimony that technology today is not yet sufficient to allow for comparisons of complex protein products. Do you agree with that?

Mr. ALLAN. Well, it has to be viewed on a case-by-case basis. I think for the product we developed the analytical methodology that we used, which was fairly extensive, was very adequate to demonstrate the structural characterization of the property.

Mr. DAVIS OF VIRGINIA. DO you think it depends?

Mr. ALLAN. It will depend on the products. There are some proteins that are fairly simple, relatively speaking, and you can characterize them extremely well.

Mr. VENKATARAMAN. I agree. I think on a case-by-case basis there are several proteins that can be characterized well today, and science continues to evolve. Academic groups and other companies I know are working very actively toward creating novel technologies to be able to do this for more complicated products. And I think a regulatory and a legal legislative incentive is going to propel that technology forward much faster to be able to do this much more sophisticatedly.

Mr. DAVIS OF VIRGINIA. How close are we, do you think? It is hard to say, I know, but a couple years, 10 years?

Mr. VENKATARAMAN. It is difficult to say, but 4 years ago, when we started working on our program, people thought it was impossible to do. We were discouraged extremely. Today we have an application, we have talked to the FDA. It has been completely solved. I think similar situations have been reported by other people. So it is a matter of providing the right incentives for the scientists to be able to take it on.

Mr. DAVIS OF VIRGINIA. OK. Are there any non-clinical tests or technologies that could fully substitute for studying the safety of biotech products in humans?

Mr. VENKATARAMAN. I would say that the safety, per se, so the comparability of the two products, characterization becomes a very important aspect of knowing how close you are to the innovator product. I think there are multiple analytical techniques that provide you very rigorous estimation of the product quality and product attributes, so yes.

Mr. DAVIS OF VIRGINIA. All right.

Let me ask Dr. Schwieterman and Ms. Gerrard, the FDA highlighted in its testimony the importance of ensuring that facilitating the development of follow-on product through abbreviated pathways doesn't discourage innovation and the development of new biological products. They also refer to the Hatch-Waxman Act as a balanced approach. Do you think an extension of data exclusivity period and certain patent protections would help encourage innovation and development with biological products?

Ms. GERRARD. I am not a lawyer. I am a scientist. I guess I have confidence in the innovation of biotech companies that I work with to continually come up with new and better products.

Mr. DAVIS OF VIRGINIA. All right. From a scientific point of view it is achievable, but from a policy point of view you are going to take a pass on it?

Ms. GERRARD. I am not a lawyer. I am a scientist.

Mr. DAVIS OF VIRGINIA. That is fine.

Mr. SCHWIETERMAN. I will take a pass, as well. I am a physician scientist. From a scientific point of view I agree with what Dr. Gerrard said.

Mr. DAVIS OF VIRGINIA. Well, Henry and I are both lawyers. Thank you.

Chairman WAXMAN. Thank you, Mr. Davis.

Mr. Yarmuth.

Mr. YARMUTH. Thank you, Mr. Chairman.

As a child I was left way behind on science, so I am going to pass on the science questions for a minute and ask something I know a little bit more about, and that is the business side of this, and I am asking business questions of a panel of scientists. I understand that.

Am I correct in assuming—and anyone can answer this—I take it, just reading between the lines, we have several representatives from generic manufacturing companies and one from a brand name company. Judging from what we have heard about the complexity of these biologic drugs as opposed to chemical-based drugs, and we all know the stories about how chemical-based drugs cost pennies apiece to produce and they are sold for whatever, but it seems to me that the economics of biologics are significantly different and more complex and therefore dramatically more expensive. If I am correct in that assumption and the process is inherently expensive, how much money can we save by producing them on the generic basis or follow-on basis as opposed to the brand name?

I guess a premise, we know that for Claritin and for Zantac and all these other products, and many of the drugs that are actually still by prescription, that we have a significant amount spent for advertising and marketing. I assume marketing, anyway, is still a big component of the biologics business. But what are we talking about, either from a historical perspective that you know about or potentially that we are talking about saving by allowing these drugs to be produced generically?

Mr. ALLAN. I can give that a shot. Actually, I don't think anybody around this table is from the generic industry. Some of us are from the innovation biotechnology industry.

With regard to price, it is going to be a case-by-case basis. There is no doubt to make a complex protein is more expensive to make than a small molecule. The manufacturing facilities that are needed, the overhead, so to speak, that goes into the whole program is probably larger than the financial commitment you would want to make for a small molecule plant. So I think intrinsically it is a more expensive business, but I believe that, you know, certainly none of us would be sitting around this table if we felt that we couldn't make these types of products at a significant price reduction to the innovator product. It will be case-by-case. What would be the percentage reduction I don't think we could—I certainly would not comment on that right now, but, as I said, it will be less expensive.

Mr. YARMUTH. Go ahead.

Mr. VENKATARAMAN. I was just going to add one comment. I don't know if I can give you any numbers, but what I do know is that the margin between the cost to manufacture and the actual price is significant. I don't have exact numbers, but it is quite significant, and I assume that could translate into cost savings in the long run.

Mr. YARMUTH. Again, I understand I am asking business questions of scientists, but would the savings result, assuming that we allow an easier pathway to producing generics, would the savings result more from the competitive aspect, or would they result from the fact that, just because we have protected the brand name manufacturer, that we have allowed that price to be very, very high, and that just by eliminating the exclusivity we bring the price down? Would the savings be inherent? Would they be related to competition, or is it just because we are allowing exorbitant profits now, understanding that those profits are being allowed to allow the company to recover some of its investment?

Mr. ALLAN. I think it will be the introduction of competition, to a certain extent.

Ms. GERRARD. And my economic knowledge might be right behind my legal knowledge, but I think what we have to understand is that, while biologics might be more expensive to make than drugs, that there is still a huge margin there, and that, while the cost savings, even conservative estimates that say 25 percent, which we have seen, when you consider that the cost of a biologic is so high that a 25 percent savings is a huge amount.

Mr. YARMUTH. You look like you want to answer.

Mr. VENKATARAMAN. The pricing for a drug that a company like Momenta would launch as a generic would be lower by at least 20, 25, 15 percent, depends on the dynamics, but because the lower prices of the drug I think the cost saving would be achieved.

Mr. YARMUTH. Ms. Mollerup, did you want to comment?

Ms. MOLLERUP. Yes. I mean, cost is an important consideration and I think that a lower cost of drugs is good, as long as it is not at the expense of patient safety. I guess, again, back to the need for clinical trials, I would like to share with you, an example which I guess indicates somewhat where the borderline may be. In Europe we have not only had two approvals of follow-ons, but also one rejection. That was on an Interferon Alpha that did not show comparability in its clinical trial in that more patients had relapse of their disease after the treatment with Alferon was stopped, compared to the reference product, and there were also more side effects in the Alferon group. Again, I am not an economist. I am a scientist, but it just goes back to the equation of cost savings, that some cost savings can be realized but the products are expensive to produce, and as this example from Europe shows, care really has to be exercised as to make sure that the appropriate comparable clinical data, not a copy of the original data set that was handed in, but appropriate comparable data ensuring comparable efficacy and safety is included.

Mr. YARMUTH. Thank you.

Chairman WAXMAN. Thank you, Mr. Yarmuth.

Mr. Welch.

Mr. WELCH. Thank you, Mr. Chairman.

Dr. Gerrard, Dr. Mollerup argued that the risk of immunogenicity from a follow-on product must always be evaluated with clinical trials. That is my understanding of her testimony. In your view, are clinical trials the best or the most sensitive method of detecting this?

Ms. GERRARD. Not always. I think we have to keep in mind that immunogenicity, as I stated, a product having greater immunogenicity really is not an issue; it is when there are clinical consequences. Immunogenicity just means you make antibodies to the product. Most of the time they are not neutralizing. Many times they are temporary. Patients continue to be treated. So it is not always an issue.

Second, is clinical trial the best way to determine immunogenicity differences between two products? It may not always be the case. Sometimes more rigorous analytical comparisons, either an assessment of the product and product instability are really a much more sensitive way of determining whether that product is going to cause problems.

Mr. WELCH. Thank you.

Dr. Schwieterman, would you agree with that?

Mr. SCHWIETERMAN. Yes, I would. I think the concept of immunogenicity is one that has been talked about a lot, but, in fact, it is a quite complex subject. There are certain kinds of immunogenicities, then there are other kinds. We have had many day-long conferences about this. The ability of clinical trials to detect immunogenicity depends on what you are talking about. For most of the things that have been bandied about, actually clinical trials are rather poor measures for picking up the kinds of outcomes that you have heard.

Mr. WELCH. Thank you.

I would ask this question to both of you, as well. Opponents of the generic biological pathway, as you know, always raise the example of Eprex, Johnson & Johnson's European version of Epogen. Can you explain a little bit about what happened with Eprex? I will start, I guess, with you, Dr. Schwieterman.

Mr. SCHWIETERMAN. I don't know, of course, the data on the manufacturing changes that were made, nor was I privy to the investigations made. I know that Johnson & Johnson underwent a great deal of investigations. I mean, just to tell the story as I know from my standpoint, Eprex, which was one of the erythropoietin—ESAs, they are called, in general, erythropoietic stimulating agents—was marketed and approved overseas, and then cases of autoimmune disease or a very bad autoimmune immunogenic reaction to the drug, itself, ensued. In other words, the body started reacting to its own protein based upon that.

The thing about this particular case that is different is that, No. 1, it occurred overseas, so, you know, there was no real knowledge of whether the analytic tests that were performed there were adequate or complete and whether they would have been picked up at the FDA.

No. 2, the ultimate investigation into this product, as I understand it from Dr. Segal's testimony several weeks ago, picked up on impurities that are actually determined with analytic tests after the fact, and most of the investigation ensued upon that; that is to say, the actual analysis of the product, itself.

From my vantage point, it is clearly an important issue, because we need to understand it, but it doesn't visciate, it doesn't make the arguments about analytic tests weaker, in my estimation. In some ways it makes them stronger.

Mr. WELCH. Go ahead, Dr. Gerrard.

Ms. GERRARD. I was just going to add to that. Pure red cell plasma is a very serious disease, but it occurred in 1 in 10,000 patients. So could this have been detected in a typical clinical trial of, say, several hundred people? No, it could not. What actually did resolve the issue for Johnson & Johnson's Eprex was a more rigorous analytical characterization to resolve that problem.

Mr. WELCH. Thank you. How large a clinical trial would have been required to identify that side effect?

Ms. MOLLERUP. I think that everyone agrees it would have taken an extremely large clinical trial, and, from my perspective, the purpose of doing these comparative immunogenicity trials where you can, from the blood samples, isolate antibodies, characterize them, find out whether they are benign or not, and I fully agree with Dr. Gerrard that not all antibody responses are a safety issue.

But with the case of these comparable clinical trials to test immunogenicity, the real important point here is that such trials can tell us if there is a major problem. For innovator products, as well as for follow-ons, it is the long-term safety monitoring that is also needed in order to pick up on minor problems like this.

Mr. WELCH. How large a clinical trial would have been required, then, Ms. Mollerup?

Ms. MOLLERUP. I don't have the clinical for Eprex because I don't have that statistic, but, back to Dr. Segal's testimony, it would take a study of about 50,000 patients to have a good chance of detecting a serious effect in a patient, 1 patient out of 1,000. But I don't have the statistics on Eprex.

Mr. WELCH. And my understanding—anybody can answer this—is that Johnson & Johnson, itself, doesn't argue that the Eprex problem would have been avoided, in fact, had they conducted a clinical trial before marketing the change product. Dr. Gerrard?

Ms. GERRARD. No, they would not have detected it in a clinical trial. Every product is subject to post-marketing surveillance.

Mr. WELCH. Right.

Ms. GERRARD. So a very rigorous post-marketing surveillance program is also important for every product.

Mr. WELCH. Dr. Schwieterman.

Mr. SCHWIETERMAN. One point I want to make is you don't conduct clinical trials for no reason. You are exposing patients to agents and putting them through a protocol and data collection and blood drawing and so forth to collect scientific data for scientific reasons that are pre-established in hypotheses, and so to argue that clinical trials should be conducted all the time is really to negate the basic premise of a clinical trial, which is the study of question.

In the case of Eprex, it would have been an impossibly large study to have studied that particular issue; therefore, a clinical trial not only would have been undetected, insensitive to that particular change; it wouldn't have offered any information at all.

Mr. WELCH. Just following on your point, would it make scientific sense to argue that the expressed example supports a clinical trial requirement for follow-on products but does not support that same requirement for brand name products?

Ms. MOLLERUP. I think, from looking at what is required for the brand name industry, I mean, the trials that we undertake, both phase two and phase three trials, immunogenicity is an obvious part of that program, because we are working with proteins and the immunogenetic profile of our products are also not established as we take them through the clinical program, so that is certainly part of the testing we do, as well.

Mr. WELCH. I'm not sure I understand you. You are saying that you have to have those clinical tests for the follow-on products but you don't have to have them for the brand name products?

Ms. MOLLERUP. No. I am saying the exact opposite. I am saying that we, in the brand name products clinical trials that we use to take these to the market, immunogenicity studies are an integrated component, and what we find reasonable to establish clinical comparability for the follow-ons is to also study immunogenicity in an appropriately sized comparative trial, and that will be a lot smaller than the innovator phase three studies.

Mr. WELCH. Dr. Schwieterman, go ahead.

Mr. SCHWIETERMAN. I guess I would disagree with that. Mandated clinical trials to study immunogenicity is not something that is scientific, but rather political. In this particular case, if the science is there, depending upon the drug, depending upon the question, the patient, and the test, you could do a clinical study in certain instances where you believed that information would be useful from that clinical study. But to mandate it for all studies would be to also perform it for those cases where it wouldn't be useful.

I think that what ought to happen is that the FDA, like they do now, be able to have the flexibility and the authority to use their assessments of the data and the context of that data to make judgments about the need for further clinical studies.

Mr. WELCH. Thank you.

Dr. Gerrard, last word?

Ms. GERRARD. I will just add to that. I think FDA does need that flexibility. You look at the history of the product, have there been any clinical consequences to the immunogenicity? What about the analytical characterization? You look at the whole picture. If there are remaining questions, of course safety is paramount. We want FDA to have the ability to request any additional data that they need to make sure that product is safe.

Mr. WELCH. Thank you. I yield the balance of my time.

Chairman WAXMAN. Thank you very much, Mr. Welch.

Dr. Mollerup, would you support giving FDA the ability to require and enforce post-market studies for both the generic and for the brand name drugs?

Ms. MOLLERUP. I am from Europe, so I have a fair amount of knowledge of the regulatory system here in the United States, but may not be accurate on all the details. From my perspective, the FDA should be able to put the same requirements to both innovators and follow-ons, because the same safety issues are involved.

Chairman WAXMAN. Right. In the United States the manufacturer agrees, when the product is licensed, to do followup tests for post-marketing, but they may not do it because there is not a sanction except to take them off the market, which has never been used. Do you think FDA should have the power to require postmarketing safety studies? You say it should be for both or either when it is necessary. Do you think FDA ought to have that power?

Ms. MOLLERUP. The power not only to ask for the data, but also actually to get it?

Chairman WAXMAN. And to insist it be done?

Ms. MOLLERUP. Yes, I think they should.

Chairman WAXMAN. Thank you.

Well, I thank all of you very much. You have been very helpful, and I appreciate your testimony. This may be self-serving, but the bill does allow FDA to require clinical trials. It allows FDA to do whatever is necessary to determine that the science indicates a generic version is safe and effective.

Thank you very much.

I want to call forward the witnesses for our third panel.

Yvonne Brown is an individual living with multiple sclerosis and is speaking today on behalf of the National Multiple Sclerosis Society.

Mary Nathan is an individual living with a rare disease called Gaucher disease, and is speaking today on behalf of the National Organization for Rare Disorders.

Nelda Barnett is a Board Member for AARP.

Priya Mathur is the vice chair of health benefits, Board of Administration, at the California Public Employees' Retirement System [CalPERS].

Scott McKibbin is the special advocate for prescription drugs for the State of Illinois.

Dr. Henry Grabowski is a professor of economics and the director of the program in Pharmaceuticals and Health Economics at Duke University.

Jonah Houts is a senior analyst at Express Scripts, Inc., a pharmacy benefit management company [PBM], representing 1,600 clients, including large, self-insured employers, government payers, unions, and health insurance companies, and covering more than 50 million people.

We welcome you all to this hearing today. Your prepared statements will be in the record in full. We would like to ask each of you to limit the oral presentation to around 5 minutes.

It is the custom of this committee, as you have already observed, having sat through the earlier panels, to ask all of the witnesses to be sworn in, so I would like to ask each of you to rise and raise your right hands.

[Witnesses sworn.]

Chairman WAXMAN. The record will indicate that each of the witnesses answered in the affirmative.

Ms. Brown, why don't we start with you, if you have the mic passed over.

The timer, by the way, will be green, and then it will turn to yellow for the last full minute, and then red when that last minute is up.

Thank you so much for being here.

STATEMENTS OF YVONNE BROWN, FOR THE NATIONAL MULTIPLE SCLEROSIS SOCIETY; MARY NATHAN, FOR THE NATIONAL ORGANIZATION FOR RARE DISORDERS [NORD]; NELDA BARNETT, BOARD MEMBER, AARP; PRIYA MATHUR, VICE CHAIR, HEALTH BENEFITS-BOARD OF ADMINISTRATION, CALIFORNIA PUBLIC EMPLOYEES' RETIREMENT SYSTEM [CALPERS]; SCOTT D. MCKIBBIN, SPECIAL ADVOCATE FOR PRESCRIPTION DRUGS, STATE OF ILLINOIS; HENRY GRABOWSKI, PH.D, PROFESSOR OF ECONOMICS, DIRECTOR, PROGRAM IN PHARMACEUTICALS AND HEALTH ECONOMICS, DUKE UNIVERSITY; AND JONAH HOUTS, SENIOR ANALYST, EXPRESS SCRIPTS, INC.

Statement of Yvonne Brown

Ms. BROWN. Thank you, Chairman Waxman and distinguished members of the committee, for inviting me to provide testimony at this hearing, and thank you, Chairman Waxman, for your leadership on this issue.

My name is Yvonne Brown. I live in Waldorf, MD. I have multiple sclerosis [MS]. I am not a pharmaceutical company. I am not a lobbyist. I am simply a 44-year-old woman who struggles every day with the devastating effects of MS and the unaffordable cost of treatment.

MS is chronic, it is unpredictable, an often disabling disease of the central nervous system. It basically stops people from moving in one way or another. There is no cure. MS causes loss of coordination, memory, extreme fatigue, paralysis, blindness, and many other symptoms. These problems can be permanent or they can come and go.

More than 400,000 Americans have MS, and every hour someone is newly diagnosed. The National Multiple Sclerosis Society recommends treatment with one of the FDA approved disease modifying drugs to lessen the frequency and severity of attacks and to help slow the progression of disability. Unfortunately, the cost is often financially devastating. I know this personally.

Four of the six FDA approved disease modifying drugs are considered biological drugs. They range from $16,000 to $25,000 a year. That is about twice the amount of Social Security disability I receive annually. For me, sometimes the financial struggle to get my treatment can be troubling, more troubling than this incurable disease.

I am here today to appeal to the committee. My personal story is an example of the immediate need for this legislation that Chairman Waxman has introduced.

In the past I have struggled a lot with my MS and with trying to get the prescriptions I need to feel a little better. I was diagnosed with MS in April 2000 at 37 years old. In August 2000, I was prescribed Avonex, a biological drug from Biogen. The cost of Avonex is high, and I did whatever I could to afford my prescribed therapy. I sold my computer, I disconnected my phone, I skipped paying a lot of my bills. Despite this, I lost my home before the end of 2001 and I was living in my car. From 2001 to 2005 I was homeless.

I struggled for years to get approval from Social Security and I tried for over 3 years to be approved for subsidized housing. I was even turned down for help at shelters because of my MS. The staff there felt that I was a health liability due to my problems with balance and frequent falls. I became accustomed to begging, borrowing, and pleading for any help so I could get treatment.

Unfortunately, access to my treatment was sporadic and I paid the consequences with increased symptoms and more frequent attacks. It was a terrible cycle. As a result of not having access to Avonex for an extended period of time in 2004 I was hospitalized. The cost of my 24 hour hospital stay was nearly $1,000. I am still trying to pay that bill.

Today, after finally being approved for Social Security disability, I receive $1,100 a month, and I am covered under Medicare. I have coverage for my medications, but my co-payment is $220 a month just for Avonex. When you only have $1,100 a month to live on, $220 might as well be $220 million.

I don't want to be homeless or live in my car again, so I cannot miss rent. I don't want to risk my health, so I cannot skip too many meals. I often skip paying bills, but I cannot get too far behind or risk losing my electricity or other vital services. And I do my best to pay my share to those who provide my treatments. Even today I must miss my treatments occasionally. There is simply nothing I can do sometimes.

It is a misconception that help is readily available. Existing programs are often difficult to navigate, have varying criteria, take a long time, and sometimes run out of money. For example, last year I was finally approved for assistance by the National Organization for Rare Disorders. Before I received my assistance they ran out of funding. It was also possible to get assistance sometimes from Biogeniodec. After asking them for help over a year ago, I think I am close to getting help with coverage during the Medicare part D donut hole, which I will already enter in April. I learned my lesson, though. This time I know not to count my chickens before they hatch.

As a person with MS, I take other prescription drugs for hypertension, depression, and several supplements. The difference is that the generics are available. This keeps my co-payments low and manageable. Most importantly, I do not have to miss these treatments because I cannot afford them. But this is not true for my MS therapies and never will be unless something changes.

Hopefully you can help with a solution. I am a person with a chronic, life-long, costly disease, but I want to stay out of a wheelchair, I want to stay out of the hospital, I want to contribute my talents to the community, I want to pay my taxes, I want to be healthy so I am able to help others who have MS. I want to stay on my treatment. If I don't have access to treatments, my health will decline.

The stress from the story I have told you, which I live with, has caused me to begin to lose my hair. Frankly, I don't really care. I just want to battle this beast that is trying to take away my movement.

My story is not unique. Millions rely on biologic drugs. Millions struggle terribly with the cost. If I can leave this committee with one thought, it is that no matter how good a drug is supposed to be, it has no chance of being effective if it is not affordable to those who need it.

For a long time no treatments were available for MS. Now there are. The sad thing is it doesn't matter. Some people just can't afford them. The cost is too much. We have to change that. This legislation has the power to move us a little closer. We all know that providing more affordable medications for all Americans is a serious priority. For biologic MS therapies, we will never, ever reach that goal if we don't start by simply providing the pathway. It is a necessary first step.

Thank you again for your invitation and attention. I hope you remember me, and people like me, as you consider this legislation. Please help provide more affordable biological drugs for those who desperately need them. Help establish a regulatory pathway for the FDA to review and approve follow-on biological therapies.

Thank you.

Chairman WAXMAN. Thank you very much, Ms. Brown.

Ms. Nathan.

Statement of Mary Nathan

Ms. NATHAN. Mr. Chairman and distinguished members of the committee, I want to thank you for the opportunity to testify before you today. My name is Mary Nathan, and I am affected by Gaucher disease.

As one of 4,800 people being treated worldwide with Cerezyem, I understand, in a very practical way, what it means to be alive because of a recombinant biological medicine. I also understand what happens when the cost of a life-saving drug is unaffordable.

Gaucher disease is a rare genetic disorder classified into three categories and characterized by the deficiency of an enzyme necessary to break down fats called glycolipids. Because the enzyme is in short supply, lipids collect in the spleen, liver, bone marrow, and other organs. Left unchecked, the accumulation of lipids causes problems such as anemia, bleeding, organ dysfunction, abdominal enlargement, deterioration of the joints and bones, breathing problems, fatigue, and reduced ability to fight common infections. Type I is the most common. It strikes 1 in 40,000 people in the general population, and 1 in 600 Jews of Eastern European origin.

When I was diagnosed in 1966 at the age of 11, very little was known about Gaucher disease. Given the increased size of my spleen and my low blood count, doctors scheduled me for a splenectomy within weeks of my diagnosis. Shortly after that I was hospitalized with a high fever, excruciating pain, and an inability to walk. We learned later that lipids had migrated quickly to my bones, since the doctors had removed my spleen. We also learned that I had experienced a Gaucher bone crisis, a painful episode that would repeat often as my disease progressed.

By the time I entered college there was little doubt that I had a severe form of what is known as Type I Gaucher disease. At the age of 23 I underwent orthopedic surgery to straighten my leg and replace my destroyed hip. After a long recovery I was able to walk without pain for the first time in years. This respite lasted until 1988, when the implanted prosthesis became painful and unstable, so again I underwent surgery and began to experience complications that left me fighting for my life.

My red blood cell count was dangerously low due to a reaction, depriving my bones of oxygen. I then began to experience an ongoing cascade of bone infarcts, vertebrae fractures, and a serious fracture of my other hip.

To head off further damage, my doctor suggested a surgery of last resort known as a girdlestone procedure to repair my hip. Few patients ever walk again after this procedure.

What happened next marked a historic medical breakthrough that would change the course of my life and my disease. After 30 years of intensive scientific research, scientists at the National Institutes of Health discovered a treatment for Gaucher disease, and in April 1991, the Food and Drug Administration approved a commercial version called Ceredase.

After 3 years of enzyme replacement therapy, my overall health improved to a point where reconstructive hip surgery was possible. In November 1994, after 7 years in a wheelchair, I took my first real steps.

There is no question in my mind that I am alive today because of the orphan drug Ceredase. What concerns many of us, however, is that the miracle drug is priced out of the reach of individuals, and thus poses unprecedented challenges for patients who need the drug, for the doctors who treat us, for employers struggling with the high cost of health insurance, and for insurers and government programs helping to pay our medical bills.

In 1994 most patients were converted to Cerezyme, the Genzyme Corp.'s newly approved orphan drug, to replace Ceredase. The cost of Cerezyme differs from patient to patient because dosages are based on body weight. My dosing regimen is 60 units per kilogram of body weight for infusion. At 130 pounds, my treatment runs about $12,600 per administration, or about $300,000 a year for 24 doses. An additional $25,000 in cost is added for administering the drug and testing and monitoring my response and overall health. This brings the cost for all charges related to my treatment to over $328,000 a year. Now, over a 16-year period since its approval in 1991, I estimate that the payments for my drug have reached well over $4.5 million.

In conclusion, the wave of the future in medicine is biotechnology to treat rare diseases like mine and those diseases affecting wider populations. There is no reason why biogenerics cannot take their rightful place in America's marketplace alongside generic drugs.

Based on some estimates, it is said that biogenerics could save between 10 percent and 20 percent. If that holds true, millions of dollars could be saved annually just for the 4,800 patients currently on Cerezyme.

Mr. Chairman, I want to thank you personally for introducing your legislation. It is time to make safe and effective life-saving biotech therapies accessible and affordable to the millions who need them.

The Access to Life-Saving Medicines Act will create competition in the marketplace and, in turn, foster innovation. Hopefully a balance will be struck that encourages innovation yet allows more affordable follow-on biologics to come to the marketplace.

Thank you for your time and attention to my testimony.

[The prepared statement of Ms. Nathan follows:]

Chairman WAXMAN. Thank you very much, Ms. Nathan.

Ms. Barnett.

Ms. NATHAN. You are welcome.

Statement of Nelda Barnett

Ms. BARNETT. Mr. Chairman and members of the committee, I am Nelda Barnett of AARP's Board of Directors. AARP appreciates the opportunity to testify in support of creating a pathway for generic biologics.

AARP has endorsed the Access to Life-Saving Medicine Act because we believe this legislation will enable the FDA to establish a process for the approval of safe, comparable, and interchangeable versions of biologics. We call on Congress to pass the legislation this year.

Biologics are used every day to treat serious diseases such as cancer, multiple sclerosis, anemia, and rheumatoid arthritis. While biologics hold great promise for treating some of the most serious diseases, these treatments can be expensive, costing tens and hundreds of thousands of dollars. Some people are fortunate enough to have insurance coverage or the means to be able to afford these medications, but many are not so lucky.

Nothing illustrates how important it is that we have a pathway to lower-cost generic versions than the stories of millions of Americans who currently cannot afford high-priced biologic drugs, such as we have just heard.

My colleague on AARP's board of directors, Bonnie Cramer, could not be here today, but she has asked that I share with you one particular story. Bonnie suffers from severe rheumatoid arthritis, and over the years has undergone a variety of treatment options, including a biologic drug, Enbrel, which has helped her. Bonnie has encountered many people who suffer from her condition who are not able to afford medication. One particular woman was so affected by the disease that her fingers were gnarled and she had difficulty walking and used all of her energy just to get through the day. This woman recounted how she was trying to find a way to get access to Enbrel but could not due to the high cost of the drug.

Bonnie tells it best in her own words. She says, ''Having lived with this disease for 40 years, I know how incapacitating it can be and how the pain can be unbearable. I know what hope biologics can give to someone whose life is affected. To know that it cannot be obtained by other people with deadly diseases is brutal. How do you tell someone that they cannot have a treatment that may alter their lives significantly?''

The astronomical cost of these drugs not only impacts consumers, but also health care payers such as employers, private health care plans, public programs such as Medicare and Medicaid. One way to control these costs is to provide a pathway for the approval of generic versions of these drugs. Any prescription drug therapy treatment must be affordable and safe in order to be effective for individuals. H.R. 1038 leaves the scientific determinations up to those who are best equipped to address them, the FDA. Common sense, alone, tells us that the agency that has the scientific knowledge to approve the brand name biologics, surely has the ability to provide a pathway for generic approval of the same biologic.

The Hatch-Waxman Act created a pathway for FDA to approve generic prescription drugs. Twenty-three years later the time has come for generic approval of biologics. H.R. 1038 provides FDA the authority to produce the safe, comparable, or interchangeable version of the biologic. Our members and all Americans need Congress to enact this bipartisan legislation this year. We are pleased to see this committee and Members from both Houses of Congress and both sides of the aisle moving forward on this issue.

Thank you again for inviting us here. I am happy to answer any questions.

[The prepared statement of Ms. Barnett follows:]

Chairman WAXMAN. Thank you very much, Ms. Barnett.

Ms. Mathur.

Statement of Priya Mathur

Ms. MATHUR. Good afternoon. Mr. Chairman and members of the committee, I commend you for convening today's hearing and for the introduction of bipartisan legislation to enable consumer participation in the biopharmaceutical marketplace.

On behalf of the California Public Employees' Retirement System [CalPERS], I welcome the opportunity to testify about this issue of importance to our members, to our State, and to our Nation.

Let me begin by introducing myself and CalPERS. My name is Priya Mathur, and I was elected by 400,000 public sector employees to serve on the board of CalPERS, to invest their $230 billion of retirement assets, and to manage their multi-billion-dollar health care program.

CalPERS' health program covers 1.2 million active and retired public employees and their families. Notably, CalPERS is the thirdlargest purchaser of employee benefits in the Nation, behind only the Federal Government and General Motors, and it is the largest purchaser of health benefits in California.

This year CalPERS will spend almost $5 billion on health benefits, or $13.4 million per day. Of that amount, CalPERS, for the first time, will spend over $1 billion on members' prescription drugs. At a time when our State is trying to expand health insurance coverage to more Californians, slow the rate of growth in health care costs, and make our health care system more efficient, the high cost of biopharmaceutical products presents an unsustainable challenge to calPERS and to our entire health care system.

CalPERS has long been a leader in implementing cost effective health care programs. Among many strategies, we have instituted innovative prescription drug benefit cost-sharing designs to maximize the use of generics and therapeutically appropriate brand name drugs. CalPERS has actually achieved tremendous success in controlling prescription drug costs through the use of generics. This has been possible thanks to the chairman, whose efforts two decades ago led to the enactment of the Drug Price Competition and Patent Term Restoration Act of 1984, what we call Waxman-Hatch.

As you well know, Waxman-Hatch gave the FDA the authority to provide an abbreviated approval process for those products deemed equivalent to an innovator product after patent expiration. Without generic substitution, we estimate that our costs would be about 60 percent higher than they are today. Generics save our enrollees and our State taxpayers hundreds of millions of dollars every year.

In spite of all of our cost containment efforts, CalPERS has seen an average annual increase of about 13.5 percent for our HMO and PPO products since 2002.

Mr. Chairman, CalPERS' spending for biotech products is distressingly substantial and rising at a rate that is significantly higher than traditional pharmaceuticals. Because of the complex delivery requirements of many biopharmaceuticals, it is exceedingly difficult to break out a stand-alone spending line for these products. However, we believe that our spending on so-called specialty drugs is a good proxy, because biotech products make up the great majority of spending in the specialty drug category.

Total spending for specialty drugs was $83.7 million in 2006, a 1-year increase of 16.9 percent, compared to a 5.4 percent increase in traditional prescription drugs. On average, spending for biotech products was at least $55 per day, compared to traditional drugs at only $2 per day.

CalPERS supports a competitive health care marketplace that leads to innovation and life-saving medicines; however, competition does not exist today because the FDA asserts that it does not have the authority to approve biogeneric products. As a result, today's biotech companies are benefiting long after patents expire and are profiting at the expense of all Americans.

CalPERS supports giving the FDA explicit authority to approve biogeneric products that are safe. Without the ability to access lessexpensive comparable and interchangeable biopharmaceuticals, CalPERS ultimately will be forced to raise prescription drug copays or raise premiums, shifting the increasingly unaffordable costs onto the individuals who can least afford them.

Mr. Chairman, before I conclude I need to address one important issue. The opponents of this legislation—as you point out, they are limited to the biotech industry—are claiming that those who support your legislation are ignoring the safety threat of bringing biogenerics to the marketplace. I want to be perfectly clear. The safety and health of our members comes first in any decision we make on any health care policy. Therefore, we strongly support providing FDA with full discretion to make the ultimate decision about whether and when any prescription drug product, be it brand name or generic, comes to market. Your legislation does just that.

Mr. Chairman, CalPERS is proud to add our support to the growing and diverse list of stakeholders who support your legislation to open the door to biogeneric competition. Thank you for giving us this opportunity.

I would be happy to answer any questions.

[The prepared statement of Ms. Mathur follows:]

Chairman WAXMAN. Thank you very much for your testimony.

We are going to ask questions after everybody is finished.

Mr. McKibbin.

Statement of Scott Mckibbin

Mr. McKibbin. Thank you, Mr. Chairman, and thank you for the opportunity to speak on behalf of Illinois Governor Rod R. Blagojevich in support of establishing a pathway for generic biopharmaceuticals.

I want to applaud Chairman Waxman for his vision, recognizing that escalating cost of biopharmaceuticals to States and consumers is creating an economic burden on Illinoisans and State budgets nationwide. These costs will continue to make it more difficult to balance cost control and access for patients to affordable, life-saving biopharmaceuticals, both in Illinois and in the Nation as a whole.

Further, I would like to recognize Illinois Congressman Emmanuel for his cosponsorship of H.R. 1038, the Access to Life-Savings Medicine Act, and for supporting these important measures.

In my present role as a Special Advocate for Prescription Drugs, I have functional accountability for overseeing prescription drug spending for the State of Illinois. I am also a two-time kidney cancer survivor, and can speak personally from experience on both the value and the cost of therapies that treat such dreaded diseases as cancer.

I want to make it clear that I have a dual role as Special Advocate. The State of Illinois, as every State, has a responsibility to ensure that prescription drug pharmaceuticals available to consumers are safe and effective, so I would like to dispense with the issue of safety as a given for the discussion of generic legislation.

While some in this debate are seeking to obscure the real issue with inflammatory rhetoric about the potential lack of safety of generic biopharmaceuticals, it is my position that this legislation authorizes FDA to take those scientifically sound steps that are appropriate to ensure the safety of generic biopharmaceuticals.

I want to focus the bulk of my testimony on the reality of biopharmaceutical costs and the value of generic competition in this arena.

Illinois is a partner with the Federal Government in providing and paying for prescription drugs. We are also responsible for providing and nurturing a sound economy in our State, one that does not allow health care costs to bankrupt our State or to negatively impact employers or the overall business climate of our State. To this end, Governor Blagojevich has introduced a comprehensive program to expand coverage to the 1.4 million uninsured between the ages of 19 and 64, and to offer relief to many of our residents who struggle every day to pay for health care costs covered under the existing insurance plans.

There is some debate as to whether the annual increase of the cost of biopharmaceuticals is 15, 17, or 20 percent, but the difference is, in fact, not material. If, as I believe and my data will show, these expenditures for products are rising at an average of slightly larger than 15 percent annually, then within 5 years what Illinois spends on these drugs today will double. That would have a dramatic negative effect. We would not be able to afford these medications.

Many States probably don't realize the depth of what they are spending now on biopharmaceuticals. According to IMS, biopharmaceutical sales in 2006 grew to $40.3 billion. While the spending has escalated, a debate over potential for generic biopharmaceuticals has spanned four FDA Commissioners, all with a variety of prioritization on how to establish a biopharmaceutical generic approval process.

States need more than continued discussion on this issue. We need action. Chairman Waxman's bill is a great first step in actually getting us on the road to creating a framework to permit generic competition and the savings it will create.

To understand the breadth and impact of spending on biopharmaceuticals for Illinois, we examined the leading products and what the State of Illinois spends on these products. The results were staggering.

For our 227,500 member employee retiree group, the State of Illinois spent $33.2 million on a select list of approximately 100 biopharmaceuticals during the fiscal year that just ended July 2006. With that trend, this represents over 12 percent of our entire cost for drugs, and is growing at an astronomical rate both on the price and the utilization side of the ledger. The ingredient cost increase was 49.9 percent, and the plan cost per member was 50.3 percent.

The number of prescriptions for this select list of biopharmaceuticals also rose significantly, a nearly 29 percent increase. For programs administered under the State Medicaid Agency, we have seen similar cost and utilization increases, but on a much larger scale. For the most recent year in which data is available, the cost of 61 biopharmaceuticals was $1,662,000, paid for under the pharmacy benefit side, and an estimated $75 million paid for under the medical and the Part D wrap-around program. The grand total exceeded $200 million a year, without trend.

Now, much has been said about the potential cost savings of generic competition. Opponents to creating a pathway for generic competition argue that the cost savings may be only 10 or 20 percent. But let's look at the worst case scenario, a 10 percent savings. If Illinois was able to reduce its 15 percent, 16 percent annual increase in spending on biopharmaceuticals by even 10 percent, then we not only extend our ability to pay for these drugs, but we also extend our ability to continue, under State programs, to provide increased access to them.

The other issue to consider about savings is this—it appears an obvious one from my perspective, but seems lost in this debate. In the past year, biopharmaceutical expenditures have increased at double digit rates. If we do nothing for the rest of 2007, we will end the year even higher expenditures associated with those biopharmaceuticals. Every day that we delay in creating a pathway for generic competition is a day of potential lost cost savings to States, to taxpayers, and to consumers. We can not afford to wait any longer to begin the savings, even if, as opponents predict, the savings would initially only be modest.

Chairman WAXMAN. Thank you very much, Mr. McKibbin. Are you just about to conclude?

Mr. McKIBBIN. I have just a few more words, Mr. Chairman.

Chairman WAXMAN. OK.

Mr. McKIBBIN. I appreciate it.

I would just like to urge Congress to approve this legislation to authorize the FDA to apply sound scientific regulatory criteria that would give Illinois and other States and every consumer and taxpayer lower biopharmaceutical products and increased access, the result from the cost savings.

Thank you, Mr. Chairman.

[The prepared statement of Mr. McKibbin follows:]

Chairman WAXMAN. Thank you very much for your testimony.

Dr. Grabowski.

Statement of Henry Grabowski

Mr. GRABOWSKI. Thank you, Mr. Chairman and members of the committee. I am Henry Grabowski, professor of economics at Duke University.

My comments will focus on the differences between generic drugs and follow-on biologics and how these differences affect the expected budgetary savings. I also will discuss the importance of data exclusivity for innovation incentives. With my colleagues, I have examined these issues in two recent peer reviewed studies. I will make these studies available for the record, along with my statement.

Based on our analysis, we conclude that the cost of entry will be significantly higher for follow-on biologics than generic drugs. We expect fewer firms will enter, and average prices will decline less for follow-on biologics. Consequently, conservative budgetary scoring is appropriate in terms of expected savings to the Government and to other payers.

Second, in designing a pathway for follow-on biologics it is also very important that Congress balance price competition and innovation incentives. In this regard, it is important to include in the legislation a data exclusivity period that takes account of the high cost and risk of developing new entities. My statement provides data from a new study that is peer reviewed and co-authored with Joe DiMasi in this regard. The cost of R&D for a representative new biologic is now over $1 billion when one takes account of preclinical and clinical expenditures, the cost of failures, the cost of capital, and process engineering, which is higher for biologics than pharmaceuticals.

So let me now briefly summarize some of the key differences between follow-on biologics and pharmaceuticals that will affect cost savings in scoring procedures.

The first is clinical trial cost. As we have heard earlier today, some clinical trial data is going to be necessary to demonstrate comparable safety and efficacy, at least for the foreseeable future. In the case of European filings, the estimates range from $10 to $40 million for preclinical studies. This contrasts with $1 to $2 million costs for bioequivalents for generic drugs.

Second is development times. Estimates from generic firms indicate development times for a follow-on biologic are likely to range from five to 8 years. By comparison, generic drugs seldom require more than a few years to do required tests and gain regulatory approval.

Third is manufacturing cost and risk. The required capital investment in property, plant, and equipment and the cost of manufacture are also likely to be significantly higher for follow-on biologics.

Fourth, there are important differences on the demand side. It is unlikely that most follow-on drugs will be designated as interchangeable by the FDA, at least not for the foreseeable future and without extensive clinical trials. As a result, we expect the physicians will initially be cautious with respect to the substitution of follow-on products. Health care providers and patients are likely to be wary until clinical experience has accumulated and shown that a follow-on product is a satisfactory therapeutic alternative to the original innovator products.

These costs and demand side differences have important implications for entry and price competition. In our research, we find the number of entrants and the priced discounts of a follow-on biologic are highly sensitive to fixed cost. As a consequence, even very large-selling biologics are likely to have only a few entrants. For markets with only one to three entrants, we project price discounts will be in the range of 10 to 25 percent. This is in accordance with European experience to date.

These differences also have important implications for scoring cost savings. In particular, cost saving estimates based on the experiences of generic drug utilization and pricing are subject to strong upward biases. A correct accounting of this and all other relevant factors would substantially lower the savings estimates in studies such as that by Express Scripts and the PCMA.

A recent analysis by Avalier Health has very different assumptions in some important dimensions, find much lower cost savings.

The remainder of my statement covers R&D costs and innovation incentives. I understand the bills under consideration have no data exclusivity provisions or patent restoration features for innovators. The fact that there is no data exclusivity provision would allow generic firms to challenge innovators' patents from the date of first marketing approval and to enter the market soon thereafter. The resulting uncertainty in IP litigation would have significant negative incentive effects on capital market decisions for private and public biotech firms with pipelines. Many of these firms are entrepreneurial in nature and have few if any profitable products.

The exclusivity period for pharmaceuticals under Hatch-Waxman is 5 years. R&D costs have increased substantially since Hatch-Waxman was enacted 20 years ago. Five years does not provide enough time for firms to recoup the high cost of discovering and developing a new medicine. Break-even returns on R&D for the average new drug and biological product now exceed more than a decade.

Since this legislation will essentially define the terms of competition between innovators and imitators for decades to come, it is critical that it maintains strong incentives for R&D investment in new biopharmaceuticals, as well as provide incentives for price competition.

A data exclusivity period of at least 10 years in length would recognize the high cost and risk of developing new biological entities and deter patent challengers from occurring and entering until a more mature phase of the product life cycle. This would also preserve incentives for the development of new indications for existing drugs and harmonize U.S. law with that of the European Union.

Thank you.

[The prepared statement of Mr. Grabowski follows:]

Chairman WAXMAN. Thank you very much, Dr. Grabowski.

Mr. Houts.

Statement of Jonah Houts

Mr. HOUTS. Good afternoon, Chairman Waxman and fellow committee members. My name is Jonah Houts. I am a senior analyst with Express Scripts. I am pleased to be here today to discuss the issue of biogenerics from the perspective of a leading pharmacy benefit management company. Express Scripts would like to thank the chairman for his leadership in introducing this legislation, which we believe will fundamentally improve health outcomes by giving patients access to lower-cost biological alternatives.

Express Scripts monitors prescription drug trends and expenditures for 1,600 clients, including large self-insured employers, government payers, unions, and health insurance companies. I would like to talk about three basic issues today. First, I would like to speak about the trend of specialty drug spending, especially biologic agents. Second, I would like to describe the tools used by the PBM industry to control the increase in cost of prescription drugs. Third, I would like to describe how we would apply these tools to biogenerics and the potential benefit to patients, plan sponsors, and the Government.

Spending on pharmaceuticals now represents 11 percent of total health care spending. Within the pharmaceuticals are specialty drugs. These are the most high-priced biologic agents, which we are discussing here today.

I brought an exhibit which may demonstrate the increased growth here. In 2006, spending on specialty drugs was $54 billion, representing 20 percent of pharmaceutical spending. The rate for specialty drugs will almost double by 2010 to $99 billion. This rate of increase is the second highest in all of the health care field, exceeded only by diagnostic imaging tests.

In total, Express Scripts manages the pharmacy benefit for over 50 million individuals in this country. Our mission is to make the use of prescription drugs safer and more affordable. To this end, we have developed sophisticated tools, such as formularies, tiered copayments, step therapies, and drug utilization management programs, just to name a few. These tools promote the most clinically sound and cost effective use of pharmaceuticals.

One of the most potent tools that we have is the promotion of generic medications. These therapies are time tested and thus are clinically effective. They also have well characterized safety profiles. The additional advantage is that they are the most affordable for both patients and plan sponsors. For these reasons, patients achieve higher compliance rates with these therapies. Utilizing programs like I previously described, our company has an industry leading generic fill rate of 60 percent.

But it is important to recognize that all of our programs for promoting the use of generics or less expensive branded medications are reviewed by our external pharmacy and therapeutics committee. This committee is made up of both specialty and general medicine doctors, and pharmacists who are not employees of Express Scripts. Safety has and always will be of primary concern to Express Scripts.

As we have stated, spending on biologic agents is increasing at an alarming rate. This legislation will allow for a pathway at the FDA for companies to bring to market generic versions of these important medications.

The PBMs have the tools to assist patients in switching to the most cost-effective biogenerics. In fact, our switching tools will be even more effective in this market because of the limited number of patients, the limited number of prescriptions, the limited prescribing community, and the potential for enormous savings. Our plan sponsors will be very motivated to have us pursue each and every savings opportunity.

We are pleased to hear the FDA today not rule out interchangeability in the future, but, regardless, if the FDA deems a product is interchangeable or just comparable, will be quite effective at working with the prescribing physician to aid patients in receiving the most cost-effective and clinically appropriate therapy.

In the realm of branded pharmaceuticals, drugs compete on their research and development and marketing. It would be irrational for branded drugs to compete on price, as they are competing within a finite group of patients, and price reductions would result in reduced revenues for all manufacturers in the class. Generic drugs, however, can only compete on price. Without this extensive research and development, the only way for a generic to capture market share is on price. This price competition benefits payers, plans, and the Government.

This historic legislation would allow patients, payers, physicians, and PBMs to work together to make these wonderful therapies more available, with improved health outcomes and tremendous

savings.

[The prepared statement of Mr. Houts follows:]

Chairman WAXMAN. Thank you very much, Mr. Houts.

I want to thank all of you for your testimony, especially Ms. Brown and Ms. Nathan. Your very moving testimony is what this legislation is all about. When drugs are miracles, but the miracles are too expensive for people, they are not going to be there for them, and that is why we need to figure out a way to hold down costs. Providing generics is certainly, to me, one of the best ways to hold down costs. Others have suggested other ideas, but competition, market forces I think do work and have worked in the past.

Ms. Mathur, I find it stunning that in California spending on biologics or specialty drugs in 2006 was $83.7 million, and that is at a cost of $55 per day, compared to $2 per day for traditional drugs. If those kinds of spending trends are maintained, what will be the impact on CalPERS and your members in the future?

Ms. MATHUR. I think we really are at unsustainable levels, and what we fear is that in the future we will have to shift more of the cost on to the member, either through increases in co-pays or by raising premiums. We have already heard stories from some of our members that, as the cost of health care increases overall, they are less and less able to afford health care, even through our program. I would hate to see some of our members drop health care coverage that is available to them simply because they cannot afford it.

Chairman WAXMAN. Dr. Grabowski asserts that the savings from generic competition in the biologics context will be modest, in the range of 10 to 25 percent. What would even those modest savings mean for CalPERS? And let me ask this also of Mr. McKibbin for Illinois.

Ms. MATHUR. I'm sorry, Mr. Chairman. I thought you were directing that to Mr. Grabowski.

Chairman WAXMAN. The 10 to 25 percent savings, Dr. Grabowski says those are modest.

Ms. MATHUR. Yes.

Chairman WAXMAN. What will that mean, however?

Ms. MATHUR. I think it would be extremely significant. I mean, the cost for some members, $300,000 a year, 10 to 15 percent or 10 to 25 percent is a significant savings. So even though on a percentage basis the savings for biotech drugs or biogenerics might be less than for synthetic drugs, it is certainly, on an aggregate total cost basis, going to be a very large number.

Chairman WAXMAN. Mr. McKibbin.

Mr. MCKIBBIN. For Illinois, Mr. Chairman, we are talking about $20 to $50 million, depending on when we start it, if we start it this year. And those are numbers that come out of the base, so, as you know, if this trend continues at 15 percent plus, we, too, like California, will reach this point where it is not sustainable, so we will either have to make those tough choices of trying to pass more costs or to limit access, which is untenable.

Chairman WAXMAN. Thank you.

Mr. Houts, one of the frequent assertions we hear from BIO, the trade association for the brand name biotech drugs, is that when a generic pathway for biologics is established we are not going to see much in the way of savings because generic biologics won't be interchangeable like they are with traditional generic drugs. Obviously, we might disagree on the number of biologics that will end up being interchangeable, but assuming BIO is correct that a high number of biologics will be just comparable instead of interchangeable, what kind of impact will that have on spending on biologics?

Mr. HOUTS. There is still a significant savings opportunity, even if interchangeability is not granted by the FDA. Managed care plans and the PBMs, a recent example would be in the statin market, where there was a high-priced, effective statin, Statin A, and then a lower-priced and still effective Statin B. While they were different chemical entities, we were able to move market share to the cost-effective product.

We were actually able to move 49 percent of the market share when they weren't interchangeable, as you will. And so there is still a significant opportunity in the area of biologics to move patients to the preferred safe, effective, cost-effective products.

Chairman WAXMAN. Well, you said it would be safe. When therapeutic switches are made, what process is in place to protect patient safety?

Mr. HOUTS. All of those decisions are reviewed by our pharmacy and therapeutics committee that I referred to in my testimony, and this is composed of specialist physicians, and other physicians to ensure that drugs in those classes will have no adverse effects on patients.

Chairman WAXMAN. Thank you very much.

Mr. Danny Davis.

Mr. DAVIS OF ILLINOIS. Thank you very much, Mr. Chairman.

Once again, let me thank you for calling and conducting this hearing. It has, indeed, been informative, and I want to thank all of the witnesses for their testimony. I especially want to echo the sentiments that you expressed, Mr. Chairman, relative to the impact of the testimony of Ms. Brown and Ms. Nathan, consumers for whom all of us work. Hopefully, as a result of their experiences and their testimony, the hearing heightens the recognition that we must do something, and do it as quickly as possible, to try and make sure that we have available the very best and the most cost effective medical care that the country can provide. So I certainly want to again thank both Ms. Brown and Ms. Nathan for being here and for their testimony.

Mr. McKibbin, let me just commend the Governor for the State of Illinois. When I see the kind of interest that Rod Blagojevich has shown relative to health care, and especially the effort to try and make sure that pharmaceuticals are available to all of our residents at a cost for which they can pay, it makes me proud to live in the State of Illinois and proud to know that he is, indeed, our Governor. Please convey that to him.

Mr. McKIBBIN. I will.

Mr. DAVIS OF ILLINOIS. If I could direct your attention to the chart located over here, which shows the five largest Medicare Part B drug expenditures in 2005— and you may not be able to see, but listed are all of the medicines listed of biotech drugs that are regulated as biologics. Spending on Epogen, an anemia treatment, alone, was over $1.7 billion, but it was actually even higher than that, because those numbers on the chart do not include spending on the end-stage renal disease, ESRD program. Three of the other drugs are also anemia treatments, and they collectively represent over $2.1 billion in Medicare spending. Remicade, an arthritis medicine, accounted for $541 million.

My question is: are we seeing those same kind of trends in the State of Illinois? And in terms of State spending, what are the five top biologics in the State of Illinois?

[The information referred to follows:]

Mr. MCKIBBIN. Well, Congressman, we are seeing those similar type of numbers, and anyone who has a television will recognize those drugs because they are fairly heavily advertised, but those five drugs on your screen, I did a quick analysis and we are talking about $23 million a year, a little over $23 million for those five drugs on your particular chart.

For us, I took a look at the top five for just our State employee retiree group, and those top five were Enbrel, Humira, Avonex—which was talked about earlier—Lantus, and Forteo. Those were the top five drugs from a total dollar amount. On a per patient basis they are slightly different, but those five drugs are our top five, and not dissimilar to your chart. In some cases the difference may be because of Medicare and where Medicare may cover, versus an employee group, but we are seeing those similar types of trends.

Mr. DAVIS OF ILLINOIS. I know that all of us throughout the country moan and groan and talk about the speculation of Medicare and Medicaid and whether or not there are going to be increases or decreases. Many of the hospitals kind of operate on shaky ground every year. They are wondering whether or not they are going to experience severe cuts.

Are they going to have to close departments or, in some instances, actually go out of business? Should we continue to see increases in pharmaceutical drug costs, what impact do you think that would have on the hospitals, for example, in the State of Illinois, as well as throughout the Nation?

Mr. MCKIBBIN. Certainly, Congressman, it could be the tipping point, and that is something that we arc vcry concerned about. I know yourself and others in the delegation are concerned, and we would urge that this legislation be passed sooner rather than later. As I said earlier, you know, every day that goes by is a day that is a lost opportunity, and it may be, in fact, a tipping point for hospitals in the Illinois, metro Chicago, and the rest of the United States.

Mr. DAVIS OF ILLINOIS. Mr. Chairman, I see that the light is on, but could I ask Mr. Houts if he could respond to that same question relative to the continued escalation of pharmaceutical costs without relief, how this will affect the Medicare/Medicaid programs, and certainly their impact on our hospital infrastructures?

Mr. HOUTS. It is not really a field of expertise for me as far as government payers. What I can say is that there is an exceptional opportunity for the Government in terms of Part B and end-stage renal disease, especially looking at those top drugs listed there, to save a pronounced amount of money. And so, as you consider this legislation, you may want to find ways to make Part B and the ESRD program more comparable to the commercially insured market and adopt some of the tools we use to manage trend.

Mr. DAVIS OF ILLINOIS. Well thank you very much.

Mr. Chairman, again, I just simply want to commend you for your insight in introducing this legislation, the leadership that you continue to provide. I have always known of your strong interest in health care. You probably would not remember it, but way back in a different life when I used to come to D.C. to lobby on behalf of the National Association of Community Health Centers, you were always the person that we felt that we could come to and get some understanding. I mean, Senator Kennedy over in the Senate and Representative Waxman here in the House, you were our guys. I want to thank you again.

Chairman WAXMAN. Thank you. Now you are one of our guys, too. Thank you for your kind comments.

I very much appreciate all of our witnesses in this panel, as in the previous panels.

I would like to ask unanimous consent that all Members have 5 days to submit additional questions for the record to the witnesses that have appeared before us today.

That concludes our hearing, and our meeting is adjourned.

Thank you very much.

[Whereupon, at 1:29 p.m., the committee was adjourned.]

[The prepared statement of Hon. Elijah E. Cummings and additional information submitted for the hearing record follow:]

INDEX

C

F

G

O

obsolete, 99
Ohio, 45, 93
opposition, 43
oral, 31, 34, 67, 84, 103, 126
organ, 130
oversight, 75, 107, 117
oxygen, 131

P

pain, 130, 133
paralysis, 128
parameter, 99
partnership, 65,78
Patent and Trademark Office, 6, 8, 18
patents, ix, 1, 2, 3, 5, 6, 7, 8, 10, 11, 12, 16,
    18, 21, 22, 25, 34, 39, 47, 49, 50, 52, 53,
    56, 57, 58, 64, 67, 71, 74, 76, 97, 135, 140
pathways, 5, 82, 83, 89, 119
patients, 11, 50, 51, 72, 76, 77, 80, 89, 93,
    110, 114, 115, 116, 122, 123, 124, 131,
    136, 139, 141, 142, 144
Paxil, 12, 32, 35
pay off, 28, 32, 33, 38, 69
PBMs, 142, 144
peer review, 138, 139
Pennsylvania, 29
peptic ulcer, 79, 89
peptide, 83
peptides, 91
permit, 68, 84, 93, 137
pharmaceutical, ix, 1, 2, 5, 6, 8, 9, 10, 11, 13,
    14, 16, 17, 18, 22, 23, 24, 25, 29, 34, 35,
    36, 38, 53, 55, 62, 64, 77, 80, 81, 82, 84,
    93, 95, 97, 98, 99, 103, 115, 118, 127, 141,
    145, 146
pharmaceutical companies, 5, 11, 29, 55, 98,
    103
pharmaceutical industry, ix, 1, 9, 10, 24, 25,
    34, 36, 80, 93, 97

pharmaceuticals, 2, 4, 5, 8, 12, 13, 19, 36, 79,
    88, 92, 95, 96, 97, 100, 102, 134, 136, 139,
    140, 141, 142, 144
pharmacists, 10, 11, 96, 142
pharmacokinetic, 106, 108, 110, 118
Philadelphia, 51
phone, 128
PHS, 83, 93, 102
physicians, 11, 109, 110, 139, 142, 144
pipelines, 140
planning, 83
plants, 89, 99
plasma, 123
plastics, 64
play, 34, 84, 114
poor, 123
population, 105, 130
potassium, 35
potato, 80
power, 16, 61, 64, 126, 129
PPO, 134
PRCA, 116
preclinical, 4, 111, 112, 139
pre-clinical, 5, 6, 111, 112
predictability, 88
premium, 76
premiums, 135, 143
Prescription Drug, Improvement, and
    Modernization Act, 9
prescription drugs, 2, 17, 32, 46, 80, 126, 129,
    133, 134, 135, 136, 141
president, 103, 111, 113
press, 75
pressure, 35
price competition, 19, 20, 29, 139, 140, 142
prices, 9, 13, 21, 23, 27, 28, 30, 32, 33, 37, 46,
    60, 61, 76, 97, 138
private, 10, 19, 29, 30, 33, 38, 77, 133, 140
private practice, 30
private sector, 33
probability, 59
producers, 23
product attributes, 119
product life cycle, 140
production, 99, 107

Q

R

S

T